LABORATORY DECONTAMINATION AND DESTRUCTION OF CARCINOGENS IN LABORATORY WASTES: SOME POLYCYCLIC HETEROCYCLIC HYDROCARBONS

INTERNATIONAL AGENCY FOR RESEARCH ON CANCER

The International Agency for Research on Cancer (IARC) was established in 1965 by the World Health Assembly, as an independently financed organization within the framework of the World Health Organization. The headquarters of the Agency are at Lyon, France.

The Agency conducts a programme of research concentrating particularly on the epidemiology of cancer and the study of potential carcinogens in the human environment. Its field studies are supplemented by biological and chemical research carried out in the Agency's laboratories in Lyon and, through collaborative research agreements, in national research institutions in many countries. The Agency also conducts a programme for the education and training of personnel for cancer research.

The publications of the Agency are intended to contribute to the dissemination of authoritative information on different aspects of cancer research. A complete list is printed at the back of this book.

WORLD HEALTH ORGANIZATION

INTERNATIONAL AGENCY FOR
RESEARCH ON CANCER

MINISTRY OF THE ENVIRONMENT
FRANCE

Laboratory Decontamination and Destruction
of Carcinogens in Laboratory Wastes:
Some Polycyclic Heterocyclic Hydrocarbons

Editors

M. Castegnaro, J. Barek, J. Jacob, U. Kirso,
M. Lafontaine, E.B. Sansone, G.M. Telling & T. Vu Duc

IARC Scientific Publications No. 114

International Agency for Research on Cancer
Lyon, France
1991

Published by the International Agency for Research on Cancer,
150 cours Albert Thomas, 69372 Lyon Cedex 08, France

Distributed by Oxford University Press, Walton Street, Oxford OX2 6DP, UK

Distributed in the USA by Oxford University Press, New York

ISBN 92 832 2114 1
ISSN 0300-5085

Printed in France

Contents

Foreword   vii

Polycyclic heterocyclic hydrocarbons considered   1

Introduction   3

Methods of degradation   5

Collaborating organizations   6

Methods Index Table   7

Method 1:   Destruction of some polycyclic heterocyclic compounds using
               oxidation by potassium permanganate in alkaline solution   9

Method 2:   Destruction of some polycyclic heterocyclic compounds using
               oxidation by potassium permanganate   17

Method 3:   Degradation of some dibenzocarbazoles and dibenzacridines
               using hydrogen peroxide and iron(II) chloride   25

Method 4:   Destruction of some polycyclic heterocyclic compounds using
               concentrated sulfuric acid   31

Appendix A: Nomenclature and chemical and physical data on the
               polycyclic heterocyclic hydrocarbons considered   37

Appendix B: Further reactions of nitrogen-containing polycyclic com-
               pounds relevant to their degradation   43

References   45

Foreword

While there has always been a widespread interest in the field of polycyclic aromatic hydrocarbons, little research was performed in the 1970s and 1980s on their aza-analogues. However, the development of analytical methods has facilitated their analysis in our environment; their occurrence in diesel exhaust coupled with the increasing use of diesel fuel has generated an increased interest during recent years, in both the analytical field and the mode of biological action of these compounds. Such laboratory work generates waste and may occasion spills, which have to be decontaminated.

IARC has for some time been running a programme, with the support of the Division of Safety of the US National Institutes of Health, to establish validated methods for destruction of genotoxic compounds in laboratory wastes, which permitted the investigation of methods for eight classes of compounds. Further support for this programme provided by the French Ministry of the Environment (contract SRETI / MERE / 88201) has now allowed the development of methods for two new series of substances, the aza-arenes and some mycotoxins.

The Agency very much appreciates this support and hopes that this joint effort will lead to the improvement of laboratory safety.

L. Tomatis, M. D.
Director, IARC

Polycyclic heterocyclic hydrocarbons considered

The following polycyclic heterocyclic hydrocarbons (PHC) are considered in this volume. The methods described for the destruction of specific compounds may be applicable to others from the same group. However, when dealing with other compounds, the efficiency of the methods should first be verified.

Compound	Chemical Abstracts Services Registry Number	Abbreviations used in this volume
Dibenz[a,j]acridine	224-42-0	DB(a,j)AC
Dibenz[a,h]acridine	226-36-8	DB(a,h)AC
7H-Dibenzo[c,g]carbazole	194-59-2	DB(c,g,)C
13H-Dibenzo[a,i]carbazole	239-64-5	DB(a,i)C

Certified reference materials for these compounds are available from the Community Bureau of Reference, C.E.C., 200 rue de La Loi, B-1049 Brussels.

Introduction

CARCINOGENICITY

The carcinogenicity of both dibenzacridines considered in this document has been evaluated by working groups of experts (International Agency for Research on Cancer, 1983, 1987) and the two compounds were classified in group IIB, i.e., the agent is possibly carcinogenic to humans.

The same classification was attributed by the experts' working groups to 7*H*-dibenzo[*c,g*]carbazole (International Agency for Research on Cancer, 1987). The carcinogenicity of dibenzo[*a,i*]carbazole has not been evaluated by these groups, but it has been demonstrated that it is carcinogenic to rats, although at lower levels than dibenzo[*c,g*]carbazole (Boyland & Brues, 1937).

ANALYSIS

A number of methods have been proposed for the analysis of polycyclic heterocyclic compounds in our environment. They include extraction in a variety of organic solvents, clean-up steps generally using liquid partition techniques and/or column chromatography and final determination usually by coupling of chromatographic separation techniques and various detection system. Table 1 summarizes some relevant publications. Polarographic reduction of a series of carcinogens, including dibenzocarbazoles have been investigated (Podany *et al.*, 1975, 1976).

Table 1. Summary of methods for analysis and detection of dibenzocarbazoles and dibenzacridines

Compound analysed	Separation technique	Detection system	References
DB(c,g)C DB(a,i)C DB(a,j)AC	Capillary GC	FID	Wilson et al. (1984) Wright et al. (1985)
DB(a,j)AC DB(a,i)C	Capillary GC for detection of Kovats and Lee retention indices	MS	Rostad & Pereira (1986)
DB(a,j)AC DB(a,h)AC	Capillary GC	FID	IUPAC (1983) Grimmer & Naujack (1986)
DB(a,h)AC DB(a,j)AC	Capillary GC	FID & NPD	Nielsen et al. (1986)
DB(a,j)AC	Capillary GC	FID & MS	James et al. (1983)
DB(a,j)AC DB(a,h)AC	GC on packed column	Flame thermo-ionic & MS	Shinohara et al. (1983)
DB(c,g)C	GC on packed column	FID	Lane et al. (1973)
DB(a,j)AC DB(a,h)AC	TLC on polyamide	Fluorescence under UV irradiation at 365 nm	Okamoto et al. (1983)
DB(a,j)AC	TLC on Kieselgel G	Fluorescence under UV irradiation at 254 and 365 nm	Sârbu et al. (1983)
DB(a,j)AC DB(a,i)C	HPLC on ODS column	Chemilumi-nescence	Sigvardson et al. (1984)
DB(a,j)AC DB(a,i)C	HPLC on C_{18} and cyano function columns	UV (254 nm)	Schronk et al. (1981)
DB(a,j)AC DB(a,h)AC	HPLC on C_{18} columns	UV (289 nm) spectrofluori-metry	Joe et al. (1986) Masclet et al. (1985)
DB(c,g)C	HPLC on ODS column	UV (268 nm)	Warshawsky & Myers (1981)

TLC, Thin-layer chromatography ; GC, Gas chromatography ; HPLC, High-pressure liquid chromatography ; FID, Flame ionization detector ; MS, Mass spectrometry ; NPD, Nitrogen phosphorus detector ; UV, Ultraviolet.

Methods of degradation

Oxidation of the four polycyclic heterocyclic hydrocarbons evaluated in this volume using 0.3 mol/L $KMnO_4$/3 mol/L H_2SO_4 was shown to lead to complete degradation in 1 hour. However, in view of the recently detected mutagenic effect of Mn^{2+} generated by this technique, the method was withdrawn.

Oxidation of DB(a,h)AC by 0.3 mol/L $KMnO_4$ does not lead to complete degradation in 15 hours. Thus, this method is not suitable for this compound.

Oxidation of DB(a,h)AC by 0.3 mol/L $KMnO_4$ in 2 mol/L NaOH does not lead to complete degradation in six hours. Thus, this method is not suitable for this compound.

Treatment of the two dibenzacridines evaluated in this volume with strong sulfuric acid was found to be inefficient. Thus, the method should not be used for these compounds.

Collaborating organizations

The methods in this document have been tested by the following collaborating laboratories and their description benefited from the work of the group.

Dr J. BAREK, Dr J. MATĚJKA and Dr J. ZIMA
Department of Analytical Chemistry
Charles University
128 40 Prague 2, Czechoslovakia

Dr J. JACOB
Biochemisches Institut für Umweltcarcinogene
Lurup 4
2070 Grosshansdorf, Germany

Dr U. KIRSO and Dr A. BOGDANOV
Institute of Chemistry
Estonian Academy of Sciences
Akadeemia tee 15
200108 Tallinn
Estonia, USSR

Dr M. LAFONTAINE
Institut National de Recherche et de Securité
Avenue de Bourgogne
54500 Vandœuvre, France

Dr E. B. SANSONE and Dr G. LUNN
NCI-Frederick Cancer Research & Development Center
P.O. Box B
Frederick, MD 21702, USA

Dr G. M. TELLING and Dr J. MILLER
Unilever Research Colworth Laboratory
Sharnbrook, Beds, MK44 1LQ, UK

Dr T. VU DUC
Institut Universitaire de Médecine
  et d'Hygiène du Travail
Rue du Bugnon 19
1005 Lausanne, Switzerland

International Agency for Research on Cancer
150 cours Albert Thomas
69372 Lyon Cedex 08, France

Method index table

METHODS RECOMMENDED FOR SPECIFIC WASTE CATEGORIES

Waste category	Recommended destruction method in order of preference[a]
Solid compounds	2, 1, 3, 4
Aqueous solutions	2, 1
Solutions in volatile organic solvents	2, 1, 3
Solutions in DMF	2, 1
Solutions in DMSO	2, 1, 4
Glassware	2, 1, 3, 4
Spills	2, 1

Methods 1 and 2 are applicable to DB(c,g)C, DB(a,i)C and DB(a,j)AC
Method 3 is applicable to DB(c,g)C, DB(a,i)C, DB(a,j)AC and DB(a,h)AC
Method 4 is applicable to DB(c,g)C and DB(a,i)C

Destruction of some polycyclic heterocyclic compounds using oxidation by potassium permanganate in alkaline solution

1. SCOPE AND FIELD OF APPLICATION

The method specifies a procedure for the destruction of DB(a,j)AC, DB(c,g)C and DB(a,i)C in the following laboratory wastes: solid compounds (6.1); solutions in volatile organic solvents (6.2); solutions in dimethylformamide (DMF) or dimethylsulfoxide (DMSO) (6.3); aqueous solutions (6.4); glassware (6.5) and spills (6.6).

The method has been collaboratively tested using 1.25 mg of solid DB(c,g)C + 0.75 mg of solid DB(a,j)AC and 5 mg of DB(a,i)C in 5 mL DMF. For these samples the method achieves >99.5% degradation.

The residues obtained from the degradation of these compounds by this method have been tested for mutagenic activity using *Salmonella typhimurium* strains TA97a, TA98, TA100 and TA102 with and without metabolic activation. No mutagenic activity was detected.

2. PRINCIPLE

After dissolution of the polycyclic heterocyclic compound (PHC) in acetonitrile, the destruction is effected by oxidation with 0.3 mol/L potassium permanganate in 2 mol/L sodium hydroxide solution.

3. HAZARDS

3.1 *From PHCs*

Some PHCs are carcinogenic, and gloves must be worn for all operations involving handling of the solid compounds or their solutions. Should gloves come into contact with a solution of PHCs, they should be changed as quickly as possible to reduce the risk of contact of PHCs with the skin. Whenever handling these compounds, it is recommended to work in ventilated enclosures. It should be borne in mind that due to electrostatic effects, PHCs in the solid form tend to disperse in the atmosphere and to cling firmly to surrounding surfaces. To reduce such problems when handling these compounds in the powder form, it is advisable to use cotton gloves.

3.2 *Others*

Sodium hydroxide is corrosive. Potassium permanganate is a strong oxidizing agent, and care must be taken not to mix with concentrated reducing agents. In the case of skin contact with a corrosive agent, wash the skin under flowing water for at least 15 min.

4.   REAGENTS

4.1. *For destruction*

Potassium permanganate	Technical grade
Acetone	Technical grade
Acetonitrile	Technical grade
Sodium hydroxide	Technical grade
Sodium hydroxide solution	2 mol/L, aqueous
Sodium disulfite $Na_2S_2O_5$ (CAS R.N. 7681-57-4)	Technical grade
Sodium disulfite solution	2 mol/L, aqueous
Cyclohexane	Technical grade
Potassium permanganate/ sodium hydroxide solution	To a 2 mol/L sodium hydroxide solution add solid potassium permanganate to obtain a 0.3 mol/L solution of potassium permanganate (Prepared daily)

4.2. *For analysis*

Acetonitrile	HPLC grade
Water	Deionized
Cyclohexane	Analytical grade
Sodium disulfite $Na_2S_2O_5$ (CAS R.N. 7681-57-4)	Analytical grade

5.   APPARATUS

Usual laboratory equipment and the following items.

HPLC system equipped with a spectrophotometric or a spectrofluorimetric detector.

Rotary evaporator.

6. PROCEDURE

Five mg of DB(c,g)C or DB(a,i)C or 1 mg of DB(a,j)AC in 2 mL of acetonitrile are completely degraded to non-mutagenic products by treatment for 3 hours with 10 mL of a solution containing 0.3 mol/L potassium permanganate in 2 mol/L sodium hydroxide.

NOTE: Under these conditions 0.5 mg of DB(a,h)AC is degraded only to the extent of 76% and therefore the method is not suitable for the degradation of this compound.

It must be noted that other components in wastes may react with potassium permanganate, turning the purple/green colour to brown. It is, therefore, recommended that the efficiency be checked using the analytical procedures described in Section 7.

6.1 *Solid compounds*

6.1.1   Estimate the amount of PHC to be degraded.

6.1.2   For each 5 mg of DB(c,g)C or DB(a,i)C or 1 mg of DB(a,j)AC, add 2 mL of acetonitrile and dissolve completely using, if necessary, sonication. Make sure that no solid is adhering to the wall of the container.

6.1.3   For each 2 mL of acetonitrile/PHC solution, add at least 10 mL potassium permanganate/sodium hydroxide solution, swirl the mixture and, if necessary, add further potassium permanganate solution to maintain the purple/green colour. Allow to react for at least 3 hours.

NOTE: During this period some splashing may occur, causing unreacted compounds to be isolated on the walls of the vessel. To prevent this, rinse the walls periodically with the decontaminating solution.

6.1.4   Analyse the residual mixture for completeness of degradation using the method outlined in Section 7.

6.1.5   Remove excess permanganate by addition of an equal volume of 2 mol/L sodium disulfite solution.

6.1.6   Discard.

6.2 *Solutions in volatile organic solvents*

    6.2.1 Estimate the amount of PHC to be degraded.

    6.2.2 Remove the solvent by evaporation in a rotary evaporator under reduced pressure (temperature of the bath $\simeq$ 40°C).

    6.2.3 Proceed as in 6.1.2. to 6.1.6.

6.3 *Solutions in DMSO or DMF*

    6.3.1 For each volume of DMF or DMSO add 2 volumes of water.

    6.3.2 Extract the resulting mixture three times with an equal volume of cyclohexane and pool the cyclohexane extracts.

    6.3.3 Proceed as in 6.2.1 to 6.2.3.

6.4 *Aqueous solutions*

    NOTE: Only trace amounts of PHCs may be present in aqueous solutions.

    6.4.1 Add enough potassium permanganate to make a 0.3 mol/L solution and then enough sodium hydroxide to make a 2 mol/L solution.

    6.4.2 Allow to react for three hours.

    6.4.3 Proceed as in 6.1.4 to 6.1.6.

6.5 *Glassware*

    6.5.1 Rinse glassware with four successive amounts of enough acetone to wet the glass completely. Combine rinses and treat as in 6.2.

    6.5.2 Immerse glassware in the potassium permanganate/sodium hydroxide solution. Allow to react for at least three hours.

6.6 *Spills*

    6.6.1 Isolate the area and put on suitable protective clothing.

    NOTE: For spills of powder, restrict circulation of air until the powder has been wiped up.

    6.6.2 Collect solid on a wet cloth or absorb liquid on a dry cloth, and immerse cloth in potassium permanganate/sodium hydroxide solution.

6.6.3   Add enough acetonitrile to completely wet the area and add an excess of potassium permanganate/sodium hydroxide solution.

6.6.4   Allow to react for three hours.

6.6.5   Absorb the residual solution with an absorbing material and test for completeness of degradation.

6.6.6   Examine the area of spillage under long-wave and short-wave UV light for absence of fluorescence corresponding to the PHCs.

7.   ANALYSIS FOR COMPLETENESS OF DEGRADATION

Several of the analytical methods referred to in the Introduction can be used to test the efficiency of destruction of the PHCs. The following HPLC method has been used to evaluate the completeness of degradation by this method.

7.1   Take an aliquot from 6.1.3, 6.2.3, 6.3.3, 6.4.3, 6.5.2 or 6.6.4 and add an equal volume of sodium disulfite solution to remove unreacted permanganate.

7.2   Dilute with an equal volume of water.

7.3   Extract three times with an equal volume of cyclohexane and combine extracts.

7.4   Evaporate to dryness using a rotary evaporator under reduced pressure (temperature of the bath $\simeq 40°C$).

7.5   Take up the residue in 500 μL of acetonitrile.

7.6   Analyse in HPLC using, for example, the following conditions:

> Column: 25 cm × 3.6 mm i.d. Partisil ODS-2 10 μ
> Precolumn: 5 cm × 3.6 mm i.d. pellicular ODS
> Eluent: Isocratic system. Acetonitrile:water (80:20)
> Flow rate: 1.5 mL/min
> Detection: Spectrofluorimetry
> DB(a,j)AC: excitation 366 nm; emission 425 nm;
> DB(c,g)C and DB(a,i)C: excitation 292 nm; emission 389 nm

8.   SCHEMATIC REPRESENTATION OF THE PROCEDURE

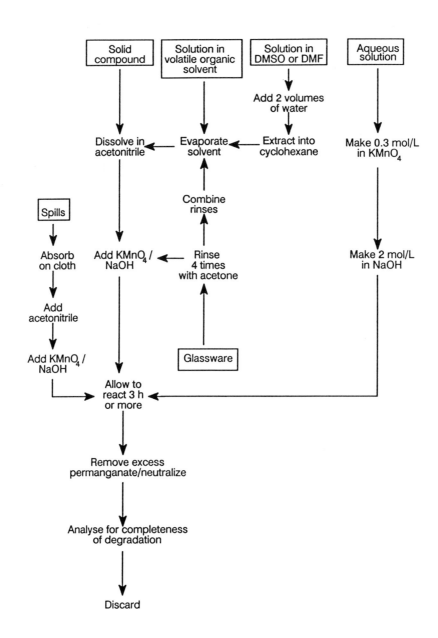

9. ORIGIN OF METHOD

M. CASTEGNARO
IARC
150 cours Albert-Thomas
69372 Lyon cedex 08
France

J. BAREK
Dept. of Analytical
Chemistry
Charles University
Prague 2
Czechoslovakia

M. De MEO
and M. LAGET
Laboratoire de
Microbiologie
Faculté de Pharmacie
27 bd J.-Moulin
13385 Marseille cedex 05
France

Contact point: M. Castegnaro

Method 2

Destruction of some polycylic heterocyclic compounds using oxidation by potassium permanganate

1. SCOPE AND FIELD OF APPLICATION

The method specifies a procedure for the destruction of DB(a,j)AC, DB(c,g)C and DB(a,i)C in the following laboratory wastes: solid compounds (6.1); solutions in volatile organic solvents (6.2); solutions in dimethylformamide (DMF) or dimethyl-sulfoxide (DMSO) (6.3); aqueous solutions (6.4); glassware (6.5) and spills (6.6).

The method has been collaboratively tested using 2 mg of DB(c,g)C and 3 mg of DB(a,i)C in 2 mL acetonitrile and 2 mg DB(a,j)AC in 5 mL dichloromethane. In these cases the method affords better than 99.9% destruction.

The residues obtained from the degradation of these compounds by this method have been tested for mutagenic activity using *Salmonella typhimurium* strains TA97a, TA98, TA100 and TA102 with and without metabolic activation. No mutagenic activity was detected.

2. PRINCIPLE

After dissolution of the polycyclic heterocyclic compound in acetonitrile, the destruction is effected by oxidation with a 0.3 mol/L potassium permanganate solution.

3. HAZARDS

3.1. *From polycyclic heterocyclic compounds (PHCs)*

Some PHCs are carcinogenic, and gloves must be worn for all operations involving handling of the solid compounds or their solutions. Should gloves come into contact with a solution of PHCs, they should be changed as quickly as possible to reduce the risk of contact of PHCs with the skin. Whenever handling these compounds, it is recommended to work in ventilated enclosures. It should be borne in mind that due to electrostatic effects, PHCs in the solid form tend to disperse in the atmosphere and to cling firmly to surrounding surfaces. To reduce such problems when handling these compounds in the powder form, it is advisable to use cotton gloves.

3.2. *Others*

Sodium hydroxide is corrosive. Potassium permanganate is a strong oxidizing agent, and care must be taken not to mix with concentrated reducing agents. In the case of skin contact with a corrosive agent, wash the skin under flowing water for at least 15 min.

4.   REAGENTS

4.1. *For destruction*

Potassium permanganate	Technical grade
Potassium permanganate solution	0.3 mol/L, aqueous. Prepared daily
Acetone	Technical grade
Cyclohexane	Technical grade
Sodium disulfite $Na_2S_2O_5$ (CAS R.N. 7681-57-4)	Technical grade
Sodium disulfite solution	2 mol/L, aqueous
Sodium hydroxide	Technical grade

4.2 *For analysis*

Acetonitrile	HPLC grade
Water	Deionized
Cyclohexane	Analytical grade
Sodium disulfite $Na_2S_2O_5$ (CAS R.N. 7681-57-4)	Analytical grade
Sodium hydroxide	Analytical grade
Sodium hydroxide solution	2 mol/L, aqueous

5.   APPARATUS

Usual laboratory equipment and the following items.

HPLC system equipped with a spectrophotometric or a spectrofluorimetric detector.

Rotary evaporator.

6.   PROCEDURE

Five mg of DB(c,g)C or DB(a,i)C or 1 mg of DB(a,j)AC in 2 mL of acetonitrile are completely degraded by treatment for six hours with 10 mL of a 0.3 mol/L potassium permanganate solution.

It must be noted that other components in wastes may react with potassium permanganate turning the purple colour to brown. It is, therefore, recommended that the efficiency be checked using the analytical procedures described in Section 7.

NOTE: Under these conditions, 1 mg of DB(a,h)AC is degraded only to the extent of ≃ 83%, and leaving the reaction overnight achieves a maximum degradation of 87%. The method is, therefore, not suitable for the degradation of this compound.

6.1   *Solid compounds*

6.1.1   Estimate the amount of PHCs to be degraded.

6.1.2   For each 5 mg of DB(c,g)C or DB(a,i)C or 1 mg of DB(a,j)AC, add 2 mL of acetonitrile and dissolve completely using, if necessary, sonication. Make sure that no solid is adhering to the wall of the container.

6.1.3   For each 2 mL of solution from 6.1.2, add at least 10 mL of the 0.3 mol/L potassium permanganate solution. Add further potassium permanganate solution, if necessary, to maintain the purple colour. Allow to react while stirring for at least six hours.

NOTE: During this period some splashing may occur, causing unreacted compounds to be isolated on the walls of the vessel. To prevent this, rinse the walls periodically with the decontaminating solution.

6.1.4   Analyse the residual mixture for completeness of degradation using the method outlined in Section 7.

6.1.5   Add sodium hydroxide to bring the mixture to 2 mol/L.

6.1.6   Remove excess permanganate by addition of an equal volume of 2 mol/L sodium disulfite solution.

6.1.7   Discard.

6.2.   *Solutions in volatile organic solvents*

6.2.1   Estimate the amount of PHCs to be degraded.

6.2.2   Remove the solvent by evaporation in a rotary evaporator under reduced pressure (temperature of bath $\simeq$ 40°).

6.2.3   Proceed as in 6.1.2 to 6.1.7.

6.3   *Solutions in DMSO or DMF*

6.3.1   For each volume of DMF or DMSO add 2 volumes of water.

6.3.2   Extract the mixture from 6.3.1 three times with an equal volume of cyclohexane and pool the cyclohexane extracts.

6.3.3   Proceed as in 6.2.1 to 6.2.3.

6.4   *Aqueous solutions*

NOTE: Only trace amount of PHCs may be present in aqueous solutions.

6.4.1   Add enough potassium permanganate to make a 0.3 mol/L solution.

6.4.2   Allow to react while stirring for six hours.

6.4.3   Proceed as in 6.1.4 to 6.1.7.

6.5   *Glassware*

6.5.1   Rince glassware with four successive amounts of enough acetone to wet the glass completely. Combine rinses and treat as in 6.2.

6.5.2   Immerse glassware in 0.3 mol/L potassium permanganate and allow to react for at least six hours.

6.6   *Spills*

6.6.1   Isolate the area and put on suitable protective clothing.

NOTE: For spills of powder, restrict circulation of air until the powder has been wiped up.

6.6.2   Collect solid on a wet cloth or absorb liquid on a dry cloth, and immerse cloth in potassium permanganate solution.

6.6.3   Add enough acetonitrile to completely wet the area and an excess of freshly prepared potassium permanganate solution.

6.6.4   Allow to react for six hours.

6.6.5   Absorb the residual solution with an absorbing material and test for completeness of degradation.

6.6.6   Examine the area of spillage under long-wave and short-wave UV light for absence of fluorescence corresponding to the PHCs.

7. ANALYSIS FOR COMPLETENESS OF DEGRADATION

Several of the analytical methods referred to in the Introduction can be used to test the efficiency of destruction of the PHCs. The following HPLC method has been used to evaluate the completeness of degradation by this method.

7.1   Take an aliquot from 6.1.3, 6.2.3, 6.3.3, 6.4.3, 6.5.2 or 6.6.4 and add sodium disulfite to remove permanganate.

7.2   Bring to pH 10 – 12 using 2 mol/L sodium hydroxide.

7.3.   Dilute with an equal volume of water.

7.4   Extract three times with an equal volume of cyclohexane and combine extracts.

7.5   Evaporate to dryness using a rotary evaporator under reduced pressure (temperature of bath 40°C).

7.6   Take up the residue in 500 µL of acetonitrile.

7.7   Analyse by HPLC using, for example, the following conditions:

Column: 25 cm × 3.6 mm i.d. Partisil ODS-2 10 µM
Precolumn: 5 cm × 3.6 mm i.d. pellicular ODS
Eluent: Isocratic system. Acetonitrile: water (80:20)
Flow rate: 1.5 mL/min
Detection: Spectrofluorimetry
DB(a,j)AC: excitation 366 nm; emission 425 nm;
DB(c,g)C and DB(a,i)C; excitation 292 nm; emission 389 nm

8.   SCHEMATIC REPRESENTATION OF THE PROCEDURE

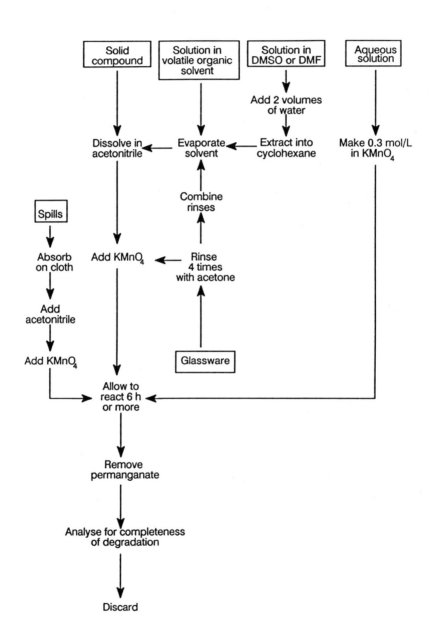

9. ORIGIN OF METHOD

J. BAREK
Dept. of Analytical
Chemistry
Charles University
Prague 2
Czechoslovakia

M. CASTEGNARO and
J. MICHELON
IARC
150 cours Albert-Thomas
69372 Lyon cedex 08
France

M. De MEO
and M. LAGET
Laboratoire de
Microbiologie
Faculté de Pharmacie
27 bd J.-Moulin
13385 Marseille cedex 05
France

Contact point: J. Barek

Method 3

Degradation of some polycyclic heterocyclic compounds using hydrogen peroxide and iron(II) chloride

1. SCOPE AND FIELD OF APPLICATION

The method permits the degradation of DB(c,g)C, DB(a,i)C, DB(a,j)AC and DB(a,h)AC in the following wastes: solid compounds (6.1); solutions in volatile organic solvents (6.2); glassware (6.3).

The method has been collaboratively tested using 2 mg of solid DB(c,g)C + 3.4 mg solid DB(a,h)AC and 4 mg solid DB(a,j)AC + 1.4 mg of solid DB(a,i)C. In these cases the method affords better than 99.9% destruction.

The residues from the degradation of all four compounds by this method have been tested for mutagenic activity using *Salmonella typhimurium* strains TA97a, TA98, TA100 and TA102 with and without metabolic activation. No mutagenic activity was detected in the residues.

2. PRINCIPLE

After dissolution of the polycyclic heterocyclic compound to be degraded in acetone, the destruction is effected by oxidation with hydrogen peroxide in the presence of iron(II) ions.

3. HAZARDS

3.1 *From polycyclic heterocyclic compounds (PHCs)*

Some PHCs are carcinogenic, and gloves must be worn for all operations involving handling of the solid compounds or their solutions. Should gloves come into contact with a solution of PHCs, they should be changed as quickly as possible to reduce the risk of contact of PHCs with the skin. Whenever handling these compounds, it is recommended to work in ventilated enclosures. It should be borne in mind that due to electrostatic effects, PHCs in the solid form tend to disperse in the atmosphere and to cling firmly to surrounding surfaces. To reduce such problems when handling these compounds in the powder form, it is advisable to use cotton gloves.

3.2 *Others*

Hydrogen peroxide is a strong oxidizing agent, and care must be taken not to mix with concentrated reducing agents. In the case of skin contact with a corrosive agent, wash the skin under flowing water for at least 15 min.

The reaction of hydrogen peroxide with iron(II) chloride is an exothermic process. Hydrogen peroxide should, therefore, be added dropwise and the reaction mixture kept in cold water or ice.

4.   REAGENTS

4.1 *For degradation*

Hydrogen peroxide (30%)	Technical grade
Iron(II) chloride ($FeCl_2$, $FeCl_2.2H_2O$ or $FeCl_2.4H_2O$)	Technical grade
Acetone	Technical grade
Sodium carbonate	Technical grade
Sodium hydroxide	Technical grade

4.2 *For analysis*

n-Hexane	Analytical grade
Cyclohexane	Analytical grade
Acetonitrile	HPLC grade
Water	Deionized
Sodium hydroxide	Analytical grade
Sodium hydroxide solution	2 mol/L, aqueous

5.   APPARATUS

Usual laboratory equipment and the following items.

UV spectrophotometer

HPLC system equipped with a spectrophotometric or a spectrofluorimetric detector.

Rotary evaporator.

6.   PROCEDURE

Five mg of DB(c,g)C, DB(a,i)C, DB(a,j)AC or DB(a,h)AC in 5 mL of acetone are completely degraded by treatment for about one hour with 0.2 to 0.3 g iron(II) chloride and 10 mL H_2O_2.

6.1 *Solid compounds*

6.1.1   Estimate the amount of compound to be degraded.

6.1.2   To each 5 mg of a test mixture, add 5 mL of acetone and make sure that the compound has been dissolved completely.

NOTE: Use a beaker of a volume at least 20 times greater than that of the hydrogen peroxide to be used.

6.1.3   Add 0.2 to 0.3 g (depending on the degree of hydration) of iron(II) chloride and place in an ice bath.

6.1.4   Add dropwise 10 mL of H_2O_2 while stirring.

NOTE: The reaction has an induction period; add the H_2O_2 dropwise until the solution boils, then complete addition over a period of 15 min.

NOTE: If the mixture does not boil, the degradation will not be complete. Repeat steps 6.1.3 and 6.1.4 with faster addition of H_2O_2.

6.1.5   Remove the beaker from the ice bath and allow to react for 30 min.

6.1.6   Analyse for completeness of degradation using the method described in Section 7.

6.1.7   If necessary, neutralize the reaction mixture by addition of sodium carbonate or sodium hydroxide and discard.

6.2 *Solutions in organic solvents*

6.2.1   Estimate the amount of compound to be degraded.

6.2.2   Remove the solvent by evaporation in a rotary evaporator under reduced pressure (temperature of bath $\simeq$ 40°C).

6.2.3   Proceed as in 6.1.2 to 6.1.7.

6.3 *Glassware*

6.3.1   Rinse glassware with four successive portions of enough acetone to wet the glass completely. Combine rinses. Then rinse with 1 volume of hexane and check for the absence of fluorescence under UV light. If fluorescence remains, repeat washes.

6.3.2   Treat rinses as in 6.2.

7.   ANALYSIS FOR COMPLETENESS OF DEGRADATION

Several of the analytical methods referred to in the Introduction can be used to test the efficiency of destruction of the PHC. The following methods have been used to evaluate the completeness of degradation by this method.

7.1 *UV analysis*

7.1.1   Add 10 mL of n-hexane to a 10 mL aliquot from 6.1.3 or 6.2.3, extract for 10 min and allow organic layer to separate.

7.1.2   Evaporate organic solvent.

7.1.3   Add 5 mL of n-hexane and take a UV absorption spectrum and compare with standards.

7.2 *HPLC analysis*

7.2.1   Take an aliquot from 6.1.3 or 6.2.3.

7.2.2   Bring to pH 10 – 12 by adding slowly, while cooling, a 2 mol/L sodium hydroxide.

7.2.3   Dilute with an equal volume of water.

7.2.4   Extract three times with an equal volume of cyclohexane and combine extracts.

7.2.5   Evaporate to dryness using a rotary evaporator under reduced pressure (temperature of bath $\simeq$ 40°C).

7.2.6   Take up residue in 500 µL of acetonitrile

7.2.7   Analyse by HPLC using, for example, the following conditions

Column: 25 cm × 3.6 mm i.d. Partisil ODS-2 10 µM
Precolumn: 5 cm × 3.6 mm i.d. pellicular ODS
Eluent: Isocratic system. Acetonitrile: water (80:20)
Flow rate: 1.5 mL/min
Detection: Spectrofluorimetry
DB(a,h)AC and DB(a,j)AC: excitation 366 nm; emission 425 nm;
DB(c,g)C and DB(a,i)C: excitation 292 nm; emission 389 nm

8.   SCHEMATIC REPRESENTATION OF THE PROCEDURE

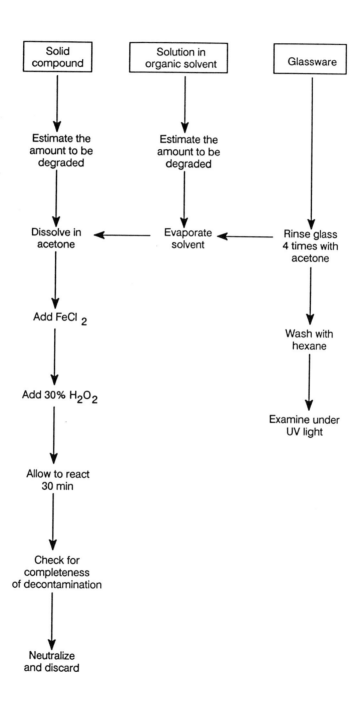

9. ORIGIN OF METHOD

U. KIRSO and
A. BOGDANOV
Institute of Chemistry
Estonian Academy
of Sciences
Tallinn, USSR

M. De MEO and
M. LAGET
Laboratoire de
Microbiologie
Faculté de Pharmacie
27 bd J.-Moulin
13385 Marseille cedex 05
France

J. MICHELON
IARC
150 cours Albert-Thomas
69372 Lyon cedex 08
France

Contact point: U. Kirso

Method 4

Destruction of some polycyclic heterocyclic compounds using concentrated sulfuric acid

1. SCOPE AND FIELD OF APPLICATION

The method specifies procedures for the destruction of DB(a,i)C and DB(c,g)C in the following laboratory wastes: solid compounds (7.1); solutions in dimethylsulfoxide (DMSO) (7.2) and glassware (7.3).

The method has been collaboratively tested with 2.5 mg DB(c,g)C and 2.5 mg DB(a,i)C in 2 mL DMSO. In this case the method achieves better than 99.8% degradation.

The mutagenic activity of the solutions resulting from samples treated by this method was determined using *Salmonella typhimurium* TA98, TA100, TA1530 and TA1535 strains. No mutagenic activity was detected.

The method has also been tested for wastes contaminated with DB(a,j)AC and DB(a,h)AC, but was not fully effective and therefore should not be used for these compounds.

2. PRINCIPLE

After dissolution of the polycyclic heterocyclic compound (PHC) in DMSO, the destruction is effected by treatment with concentrated sulfuric acid.

3. HAZARDS

3.1 *From PHCs*

Some PHCs are carcinogenic, and gloves must be worn for all operations involving handling of the solid compounds or their solutions. Should gloves come into contact with a solution of PHCs, they should be changed as quickly as possible to reduce the risk of contact of PHCs with the skin. Whenever handling these compounds, it is recommended to work in ventilated enclosures. It should be borne in mind that due to electrostatic effects, PHCs in the solid form tend to disperse in the atmosphere and to cling firmly to surrounding surfaces. To reduce such problems when handling these compounds in the powder form, it is advisable to use cotton gloves.

3.2 *Others*

Potassium hydroxide and concentrated sulfuric acid are corrosive. In the case of skin contact with a corrosive agent, wash the skin under flowing water for at least 15 min.

The addition of concentrated sulfuric acid to DMSO or water is extremely exothermic. Always add the acid to the water, and remove heat by cooling in a cold-water bath. Never add water to concentrated sulfuric acid.

4. REAGENTS

4.1 *For degradation*

Sulfuric acid	Specific gravity, 1.84 (about 18 mol/L)
Dimethylsulfoxide	Technical grade
Potassium hydroxide	Technical grade
Potassium hydroxide solution	10 mol/L, aqueous

4.2 *For analysis*

Potassium hydroxide	Analytical grade
Potassium hydroxide solution	10 mol/L, aqueous
Cyclohexane	Analytical grade
Sodium sulfate	Analytical grade, anhydrous
Acetonitrile	HPLC grade
Water	Deionized

5. APPARATUS

Usual laboratory equipment and the following items:

GC equipment or HPLC system fitted with a spectrophotometric or a spectro-fluorimetric detector.

6. PROCEDURE

Ten mL concentrated sulfuric acid will degrade 5 mg DB(c,g)C or DB(a,i)C dissolved in 2 mL DMSO in 2 h.

NOTE 1:   The efficiency of the destruction depends upon the ratio of sulfuric acid: DMSO; this should not be less than 5:1.

NOTE 2:   For the compounds tested, 2 h was found to be a satisfactory reaction time. When using this method to degrade other PHCs it should be ascertained that this reaction time is long enough to give complete destruction. If it is not, then experiments should be conducted to determine a satisfactory reaction rime.

6.1 Solid compounds

6.1.1   Estimate the amount of compound to be degraded.

6.1.2   For each 5 mg, add 2 mL of DMSO, and dissolve completely. Make sure that no solid is adhering to the walls of the container.

6.1.3. For each 2 mL of DMSO, add 10 mL of concentrated sulfuric acid; swirl the mixture, and allow to react for at least two hours.

NOTE: The addition of concentrated sulfuric acid to DMSO is a very exothermic process.

6.1.4   Analyse the residual mixture for completeness of degradation, using the method outlined in Section 7.

6.1.5   Place a vessel containing cold water (about three times the volume of the residual mixture) in an ice bath, and carefully add the residual mixture. Neutralize by addition of a cold 10 mol/L potassium hydroxide solution, and discard.

6.2 Solutions in DMSO

6.2.1   Estimate the amount of compound to be degraded.

6.2.2   Dilute the DMSO, if necessary, so that the concentration of the compound does not exceed 2.5 mg per mL of DMSO.

6.2.3   Proceed as in 6.1.3 to 6.1.5.

6.3 Glassware

6.3.1   Add a measured amount of DMSO sufficient to wet the surface of the glass.

6.3.2   Add concentrated sulfuric acid to obtain a ratio of sulfuric acid: DMSO of 5:1.

6.3.3   Allow to react for two hours, with occasional swirling.

6.3.4   If it is desired to check for completeness of decontamination, transfer residual solution to another vessel, allowing complete drainage, and analyse following the procedure outlined in Section 7. Then rinse the flask with acetone and analyse the rinse.

6.3.5   If it is not desired to check for completeness of decontamination, treat the solution as in 6.1.5.

7.   ANALYSIS FOR COMPLETENESS OF DEGRADATION

7.1   *Gas chromatography analysis*

7.1.1   Place a vessel containing about 15 mL of cold water in an ice bath and carefully add 5 mL of the residual mixture. Make alkaline (pH $\simeq$ 10) by slow addition of 10 mol/L potassium hydroxide solution and dilute by adding about 50 mL of water.

7.1.2   Extract three times with 10 mL of cyclohexane and combine the extracts.

7.1.3   Dry the extracts over anhydrous sodium sulfate. Transfer the dried extracts to a suitable flask.

7.1.4   Remove the solvent from the combined extracts by evaporation in a rotary evaporator, under reduced pressure (temperature of the bath $\simeq$ 40°C).

7.1.5   Take up the residue in about 0.5 mL of cyclohexane for analysis.

NOTE: It may be necessary to include a clean-up step on silica gel before analysing by gas chromatography.

7.1.6   Analyse by GC using, for example, a 1.8 m × 2 mm i.d. column packed with 3% OV-1 on 80/100 Supelcoport, an injection temperature of 300°C, a flame ionization detector temperature of 300°C, and an oven temperature of 260°C.

7.2   *HPLC analysis*

7.2.1   Place the vessel containing about 15 mL of cold water in an ice bath and carefully add 5 mL of residual mixture. Neutralize (pH 6 − 8) by addition of 10 mol/L potassium hydroxide.

7.2.2   Analyse by HPLC using, for example, the following conditions:

Column: 25 cm × 3.6 mm i.d. Partisil ODS-2 10 μ
Precolumn: 5 cm × 3.6 mm i.d. pellicular ODS
Eluent: Isocratic system. Acetonitrile: water (80.20)
Flow rate: 1.5 mL/min

Detection: Spectrofluorimetry
DB(a,j)AC: excitation 366 nm; emission 425 nm
DB(c,g)C and DB(a,i)C: excitation 292 nm; emission 389 nm

8.   SCHEMATIC REPRESENTATION OF THE PROCEDURE

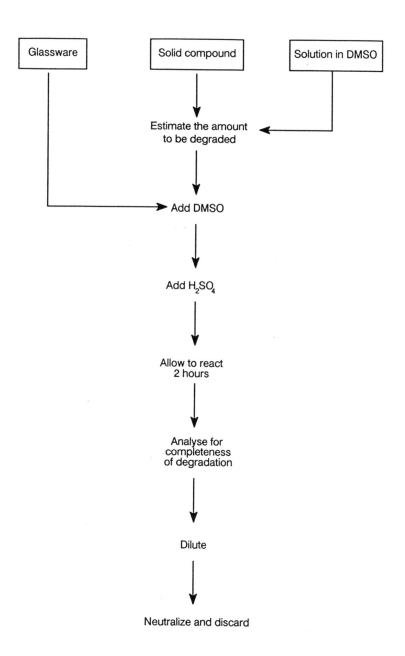

9.   ORIGIN OF METHOD

G. LUNN and E. B. SANSONE
NCI-Frederick Cancer Research and Development Center
P.O. Box B
Frederick, MD, USA
Contact point: E. B. Sansone

Appendix A

Nomenclature and chemical and physical data
on the polycyclic heterocyclic hydrocarbons considered

1. Dibenz[*a,j*]acridine

Nomenclature

Chemical Abstracts Services Registry Number: 224-42-0

IUPAC name: Dibenz[*a,j*]acridine

Chemical Abstracts Name: Dibenz(a,j)acridine

Synonyms: 7-azadibenz(a,j)anthracene; DB[*c,j*]AC; 1,2:7,8-dibenzacridine; 1,2,7,8-dibenzacridine; 3,4,5,6-dibenzacridine; dibenz(a,f)acridine; dibenzo(a,j) acridine; 3:4-6:7-dinaphthacridine; β-naphthacridine; 1.2.1'.2'-dinaphthacridine.

Molecular and structural information

Molecular formula: $C_{21}H_{13}N$

Molecular weight: 279.4

Structural formula:

Physical properties

Description:	Straw-coloured yellow needles from alcohol (quick precipitation) or amber-coloured prisms from ethyl acetate, acetone or benzene (slow precipitation) (Morgan, 1898). Light yellow needles or plates (Blout & Corley, 1947). Nearly colourless massive plates or prisms (Schoen & Laskowska, 1965)
Melting point:	216°C (Möhlau & Haase, 1902; Ullmann & Fetvadjian, 1903; Blout & Corley, 1947; Buu-Hoi *et al.*, 1955, 1966); 215-221°C (Robinson, 1973); 216-217°C (Schoen & Laskowska, 1965); 217°C (Saito *et al.*, 1956); 215.5°C (Senier & Goodwin, 1902)
Solubility:	Sparingly soluble in benzene, soluble in ethanol and acetone (Lacassagne *et al.*, 1956); dichloromethane (Kitahara *et al.*, 1978, Nielsen *et al.*, 1986); chloroform (Clin & Lemanceau, 1970a, b); toluene and trichlorotrifluoroethane (IUPAC, 1983); DMSO (Ho *et al.*, 1981); cyclohexane (Grimmer & Naujack, 1986). Sparingly soluble in alcohol and soluble in chloroform, ether, benzene or light petroleum (Senier & Goodwin, 1902)
Spectral data:	UV spectra in 36% formic acid and 95% ethanol have been published (Felton & Timmis, 1954). The following spectrum in cyclohexane has been studied by Jacob *et al.* (1984). λ_{max} (log ε) 213 (3.05), 224 (5.7), 236 (2.7), 255 (3.15), 270 (2.9), 293 (7.6), 300 (5.95), 320 (1.2), 334 (1.05), 352 (0.6), 362 (0.3), 371 (1.5), 381 (0.45), 391 (2.5).
	Infrared spectra have been reported (Pouchert, 1970). Mass spectra have been reported (Royal Society of Chemistry, 1983a; James *et al.*, 1983). The NMR spectrum has been studied by Clin & Lemanceau (1970a, b)

2. Dibenz[*a,h*]acridine

Nomenclature

Chemical Abstracts Services Registry Number: 226-36-8

Chemical Abstracts Name: Dibenz(a,h)acridine

IUPAC name: Dibenz[*a,h*]acridine

Synonyms: 7-Azadibenz(*a,h*)anthracene; 1,2:5,6-dibenzacridine; dibenz(a,d) acridine; 1,2,5,6-dibenzacridine; 1,2,5,6-dibenzoacridine; DB(a,h)AC; 1,2,5,6-dinaphthacridine; 1.2.2′.1′-dinaphthacridine; 3,4,7,8-dibenzacridine.

Molecular and structural information

Molecular formula: $C_{21}H_{13}N$

Molecular weight: 279.4

Structural formula:

Physical properties

Description:	Yellow crystals
Melting point:	226°C (Karcher *et al.*, unpublished results)
	228°C (Ullmann & Fetvadjian, 1903; Senier & Austin, 1906; Schoen & Bogdanowicz, 1960; Robinson, 1973)
Solubility:	Soluble in a number of halogenated solvents: trichlorotrifluoroethane (IUPAC, 1983), dichloromethane (Nielsen *et al.*, 1986)
	Soluble in toluene (IUPAC, 1983; Nielsen *et al.*, 1986), acetone (Lacassagne, 1956), cyclohexane (Grimmer & Naujack, 1986).
Spectral data:	UV spectra in 36% formic acid and 95% ethanol have been published (Felton & Timmis, 1954). The following spectrum in cyclohexane has been studied by Karcher *et al.* (unpublished data). λ_{max} (log ε) 219 (5.2), 224 (3.7), 246 (2.1), 258 (2.1), 267 (3.0), 287 (9.0), 295 (11.07), 316 (2.5), 330 (1.2), 344 (0.6), 353 (0.5), 363 (0.3), 372 (1.8), 382 (0.45), 392 (3.0)
	The fluorescence spectrum has been investigated (Schoental & Scott, 1949)

3. Dibenzo[*c,g*]carbazole

Nomenclature

Chemical Abstracts Services Registry Number: 194-59-2

Chemical Abstracts Name: 7*H*-Dibenzo(c,g)carbazole

IUPAC name: 7*H*-Dibenzo[*c,g*]carbazole

Synonyms: 7-Aza-7*H*-dibenzo(c,g)fluorene; 3,4,5,6-dibenzocarbazole; 1,1′-dinaphtho-2,2′-carbazol; *S*-1:2-dinaphthocarbazole

Molecular and structural information

   Molecular formula: $C_{20}H_{13}N$

   Molecular weight: 267.3

   Structural formula:

Physical properties

Description:	Yellowish needles from light petroleum of rhomboidal laminae from petroleum/acetone (Japp & Maitland, 1903); fine yellowish prisms from benzene – ligroin (Buu-Hoï *et al.*, 1949)
Melting point:	154°C (Buu-Hoï *et al.*, 1949), 158°C (Jacob *et al.*, 1986), 155°C (Japp & Maitland, 1903; Bucherer & Schmidt, 1909)
Solubility:	Soluble in ethanol (Parks *et al.*, 1986), acetone (Perin *et al.*, 1981)
Spectral data:	Fluorescence spectrum has been reported: in cyclohexane (excitation maxima at 280, 305, 335, 350 and 365 nm and emission at 363, 382, 400 and 424 nm) (Van Duuren *et al.*, 1960); ethanol (Bevan *et al.*, 1981). X-ray excited optical luminescence spectrum has been published (Woo *et al.*, 1980). Mass spectral data have been published (Royal Society of Chemistry, 1983b). The UV spectrum has been reported by Gubergrits *et al.* (1980) and Jacob *et al.* (1986). λ_{max} (log ε) 221 (4.67), 228 (4.56), 238 (4.52), 250 (4.27), 274 (4.53), 287 (4.12), 300 (4.29), 330 (3.91), 344 (4.31), 362 (4.54)

4. Dibenzo[*a,i*]carbazole

Nomenclature

Chemical Abstracts Services Registry Number: 239-64-5

Chemical Abstracts Name: 13*H*-Dibenzo(a,i)carbazole

Synonyms: 1,2:7,8-dibenzocarbazole; 13-aza-13H-dibenzo(a,i)fluorene; 1,2,7,8-dibenzocarbazole; 1,2'-dinaphtho-2,1'-carbazole; 1:1'-imino-2:2'-dinaphthyl; dinaphthylcarbazole; dinaphthyleneimine

Molecular and structural information

Molecular formula: $C_{20}H_{13}N$

Molecular weight: 267.3

Structural formula:

Physical properties

Description:	Colourless leaflets from glacial acetic acid (Cumming & Howie, 1932). Yellowish needles from benzene which give brown-red halochromic coloration with sulfuric acid (Buu-Hoï *et al.*, 1949)
Melting point:	231°C (Bucherer & Schmidt, 1909); 221°C (Cumming & Howie, 1932); 216°C (Hodgson & Habeshaw, 1947); 212°C (Buu-Hoï *et al.*, 1949), 223.5 – 224°C (Buckingham, 1982); 220 – 221°C (Lenga, 1985)
Solubility:	Sparingly soluble in acetic acid, fairly readily soluble in alcohol and in benzene, slightly soluble in light petroleum (Cumming & Howie, 1932)
Spectral data:	X-ray excited optical luminescence spectrum has been published (Woo *et al.*, 1980). Low-temperature luminescence

spectrum of dibenzocarbazoles in n-decane has been studied (Garrigues *et al.*, 1984). The UV spectrum has been reported (Felton, 1952) and Gubergrits *et al.* (1980). λ_{max} (log ε): 224.8 (4.54), 258.3 (4.47), 288.7 (4.87), 321.3 (4.22), 335.1 (4.17), 349.2 (4.01)

Further reactions of nitrogen-containing polycyclic compounds relevant to their degradation

1. Biochemical and biological methods

Table 2. Metabolic reactions of PHCs

Compound	Reaction products	Method	Reference
DB(a,h)AC	*Trans*-10,11-Dihydroxy-10,11-dihydrodibenz-[*a,h*]acridine	Incubation with rat liver microsomes	Kumar (1985)
DB(c,g)C	5-OH, 3-OH and 2-OH DBC (in decreasing order of occurrence)	Incubation with rat or mouse liver microsomes	Perin *et al.* (1981)

2. Chemical methods

Table 3 presents data from studies on the stability and chemical reactions of nitrogen-containing polycyclic compounds that have been reported in the literature and may be relevant to the establishment of degradation techniques.

Table 3. Major reactions of PHCs relevant to degradation

Compound	Reaction products	Reaction	Reference
DB(a,j)AC	A mixture of di- (24%) and tetra- (11%) aldehyde	Ozonization in dichloromethane at —30 to —50°C followed by treatment with potassium iodide.	Kitahara *et al.* (1978)
DB(a,h)AC	DB(a,h)AC-12,13-oxide	Oxidation with *m*-chloroperoxybenzoic acid in mixture of dichloromethane and aqueous sodium bicarbonate.	Ishikawa *et al.* (1977)
DB AC	Morgan's base	Reduction by sodium and amyl alcohol.	Morgan (1898)
DB(a,j)AC	9,10-Dihydrodibenz-acridine	Reduction by zinc dust in hydrochloric acid.	Blout & Corley (1947)
	N-Acetyl-9,10-dihydro-dibenzacridine	Reflux in a mixture containing acetic anhydride, zinc dust and acetic acid.	
DB(a,h)AC	Bisdinaphthacridine hexabromide	Precipitation by bromine in chloroform solution.	Senier & Austin (1906)
DB(a,h)AC	$C_{42}H_{32}O_2N_2Cl_6Pt$	Precipitation by addition of platinic chloride to a solution in alcohol/hydrochloric acid.	Senier & Austin (1906)
DB(a,i)C		Bright red compound obtained by addition of sulfuric acid, which turns dark green after addition of concentrated nitric acid.	Cumming & Howie (1932)
DB(a,i)C DB(c,g)C		The rate constants for both photodecomposition and γ-radiation-initiated oxidation have been calculated.	Gubergrits *et al.* (1980) Paalme *et al.* (1982)
DB(a,i)C DB(c,g)C DB(a,h)AC DB(a,j)AC		Frequency of S_1-S_0 electronic transitions may be applied in characterizing the reactivity of these compounds in the liquid-phase photo-initiated oxidation process.	Gubergrits *et al.* (1987)
DB(a,j)AC DB(a,h)AC DB(c,g)C		Polarographic halfwave potential has been investigated. The carbazoles are more easily oxidized than acridines.	Uibopuu *et al.* (1987)

References

Bevan, D.R., Riemer, S.C. & Lakowicz, J.R. (1981) Transfer of polynuclear aromatic hydrocarbons from particulate matter to membranes measured by fluorescence spectroscopy. In: Cooke, M. & Dennis, A.J., eds, *Polynuclear Aromatic Hydrocarbons: Chemical Analysis and Biological Fate* (Proceedings of the Fifth International Symposium), Columbus, OH, Battelle Press, pp. 603-614.

Blout, R.E. & Corley, R.S. (1947) The reaction of β-naphthol, β-naphthylamine and formaldehyde. III. The dibenzacridine products. *J. Am. Chem. Soc.*, **69**, 763-769.

Boyland, E. & Brues, A.M. (1937) The carcinogenic action of dibenzocarbazoles. *Proc. Roy. Soc. London* B, **122**, 429-441.

Bucherer, H.T. & Schmidt, M. (1909) Über die Einwirkung schwefligsaurer auf aromatische Amino- und Hydroxylverbindungen. *J. Prakt. Chem.*, **79**, 369-417.

Buckingham, J., ed. (1982) *Dictionary of Organic Compounds*, 5th edition, Vol. 2, London, New York, Chapman & Hall, p. 1595.

Buu-Hoi, N.P., Hoán, N. & Khoï, H. (1949) Carcinogenic derivatives of carbazole. I. The synthesis of 1,2,7,8-, 1,2,5,6- and 3,4,5,6-dibenzocarbazoles and some of their derivatives. *J. Org. Chem.*, **14**, 492-497.

Buu-Hoi, N.P., Royer, R. & Hubert-Habart, M. (1955) Carcinogenic nitrogen compounds. Part XVII. The synthesis of angular benzacridines. *J. Chem. Soc.*, 1082-1084.

Buu-Hoi, N.P., Jacquignon, P., Dufour, M. & Mangane, M. (1966) Carcinogenic nitrogen compounds. Part LIV. Some limitations to the Bernthsen synthesis of meso-substituted benzacridines. *J. Chem. Soc.*, Part C, 1792-1794.

Clin, B. & Lemanceau, B. (1970a) Résonance magnétique nucléaire appliquée. Analyse directe du spectre de résonance magnétique nucléaire de la dibenzo-a-j-acridine. *C.R. Acad. Sci., Paris*, **270**, série C, 598-601.

Clin, B. & Lemanceau, B. (1970b) Étude par résonance magnétique nucléaire d'isomères cancérogènes et non cancérogènes (dibenzacridines et dibenzanthracènes). *C.R. Acad. Sci., Paris*, **271** série D, 788-790.

Cumming, W.M. & Howie, G. (1932) Some dinaphthyl bases. Part 1. Synthesis and properties. *J. Chem. Soc.*, 528-534.

Felton, D.G.I. (1952) The influence of structure on the ultra-violet absorption spectra of heterocyclic systems. Part III. Some dibenzocarbazoles. *J. Chem. Soc.*, 1668-1670.

Felton, D.G.I. & Timmis, G.M. (1954) The reaction between NN-di-2'-chloroalkyl-2-naphthylamines and 4-amino-5-nitrosopyrimidines. *J. Chem. Soc.*, 2881-2886.

Garrigues, P., Dorbon, M., Schmitter, J.M. & Ewald, M. (1984) Specific identification of isomeric compounds in carbazoles series by high resolution spectrometry (Shpol'skii effect) at 15K. In: Cooke, M. & Dennis, A.J., eds, *Polynuclear Aromatic Hydrocarbons: Mechanisms, Methods and Metabolism*, Columbus, OH, Battelle Press, pp. 451-461.

Grimmer, G. & Naujack, K.W. (1986) Gas-chromatographic profile analysis of basic nitrogen-containing aromatic compounds (azaarenes) in high protein food. *J. Ass. Offic. Analyt. Chem.*, **69**, 537-541.

Gubergrits, M., Paalme, L., Uibopuu, H., Pahapill, J., Perin-Roussel, O., Perin, F. & Jacquignon, P. (1980) About the initiated oxidation of some dibenzocarbazoles. *Eesti NSV Teaduste Akadeemia Toimetised*, **29**, 305-308.

Gubergrits, M., Paalme, L., Pahapill, J. & Jacquignon, P. (1987) Polynuclear heterocyclic hydrocarbons. II: Frequency of S_1-S_0 transitions. *J. Gen. Chem.*, **57**, 2763-2766.

Ho, C.H., Clark, B.R., Guerin, M.R., Barkenbus, B.D., Rao, T.K. & Epler, J.L. (1981) Analytical and biological analyses of test materials from synthetic fuel technologies. IV. Studies of chemical structure-mutagenic activity relationships of aromatic nitrogen compounds relevant to synfuels. *Mutat. Res.*, **85**, 335-345.

Hodgson, H.H. & Habeshaw, J. (1947) The reduction of 1:1'-azonaphthalene and of some 4:4'-derivatives. *J. Chem. Soc.*, 77-78.

International Agency for Research on Cancer (1983) *IARC Monographs on the Evaluation of Carcinogenic Risk of Chemicals to Humans*, Volume 32: *Polynuclear Aromatic Compounds*, Part I, *Chemical, Environmental and Experimental Data*, Lyon.

International Agency for Research on Cancer (1987) *IARC Monographs on the Evaluation of Carcinogenic Risk of Chemicals to Humans*, Supplement 7, *Overall Evaluations of Carcinogenicity: an Updating of IARC Monographs, Volumes 1 to 42*, Lyon.

Ishikawa, K., Charles, H.C. & Griffin, G.W. (1977) Direct peracid oxidation of polynuclear hydrocarbons to arene oxides. *Tetrahedron Lett.*, 427.

IUPAC (1983) Recommended method for the gas chromatographic profile analysis of basic *N*-containing aromatic components (azaarenes) in high protein foods. *Pure Appl. Chem.*, **55**, 2067-2071.

Jacob, J., Karcher, W., Belliardo, J.J. & Wagstaffe, P.J. (1986) Polycyclic aromatic compounds of environmental and occupational importance. Their occurrence, toxicity and the development of high purity certified reference materials. *Fresenius Z. Anal. Chem.*, **323**, 1-10.

Jacob, J., Karcher, W. & Wagstaffe, P.J. (1984) Polycyclic aromatic compounds of environmental and occupational importance. Their occurrence, toxicity and the development of high purity certified reference materials. Part I. *Fresenius Z. Anal. Chem.*, **317**, 101-114.

James, R.H., Dillon, H.K. & Miller, H.C. (1983) Survey methods for the determination of principal organic hazardous constituents (POHCs) I. Methods for laboratory analysis. EPA-600/9-83-003, pp. 159-173.

Japp, F.R. & Maitland, W. (1903) Formation of carbazoles by interaction of phenols, in the orthoketonic form, with arylhydrazines. *J. Chem. Soc.*, 267-276.

Joe, F.L., Jr, Salemme, J. & Fazio, T. (1986) Liquid chromatographic determination of basic nitrogen-containing polynuclear aromatic hydrocarbons in smoked food. *J. Ass. Offic. Analyt. Chem.*, **69**, 218-222.

Kermack, W.O., Slater, R.H. & Spragg, W.T. (1930) Certain quinoline and benzacridine derivatives yielding coloured adsorption compounds with iodine. *Proc. Roy. Soc. Edinburgh*, **50**, 243-261.

Kitahara, Y., Okuda, H., Shudo, K., Okamoto, T., Nagao, M., Seino, Y. & Sugimura, T. (1978) Synthesis and mutagenicity of 10-azabenzo[a]pyrene-4,5-oxide and other pentacyclic aza-arene oxides. *Chem. Pharm. Bull.*, **26**, 1950-1953.

Kumar, S. (1985) Synthesis of trans-10-11-dihydroxy-10,11-dihydrodibenz(a,h)-acridine and its diastereomeric epoxides. Possible carcinogenic metabolites of dibenz(a,h)acridine. *J. Org. Chem.*, **50**, 3070-3073.

Lacassagne, A., Buu-Hoi, N.P., Daudel, R. & Zajdela, F. (1956) The relation between carcinogenic activity and physical and chemical properties of angular benzoacridines. In: Greenstein, J.P. & Haddow, A., eds., *Advances in Cancer Research*, Vol. 4, New York, Academic Press, pp. 315-360.

Lane, D.A., Moe, H.K. & Katz, M. (1973) Analysis of polynuclear aromatic hydrocarbons, some heterocyclics and aliphatics with a single gas chromatograph column. *Analyt. Chem.*, **45**, 1776-1778.

Lenga, R.E., ed. (1985) *The Sigma Aldrich Library of Chemical Safety Data*, St Louis, MO, Sigma Aldrich, p. 573.

Masclet, P., Bresson, M.A., Beyne, S. & Mouvier, G. (1985) Analyse rapide et sans préparation des dérivés azotés des HAP dans les aérosols atmosphériques. *Analusis*, **13**, 401-405.

Möhlau, R. & Haase, O. (1902) Ueber Naphtacridin. *Chem. Ber.*, **35**, 4164-4172.

Morgan, G.T. (1898) Action of formaldehyde on amines of the naphthalene series. Part 1. *J. Chem. Soc.*, **73**, 536-554.

Nielsen, T., Clausen, P. & Palgren Jensen, F. (1986) Determination of basic azaarenes and polynuclear aromatic hydrocarbons in airborne particulate matter by gas chromatography. *Analyt. Chim. Acta*, **187**, 223-231.

Okamoto, Y., Tsuchiya, Y., Shinohara, R. & Takeshita, R. (1983) Separation of azaarenes by polyamide thin layer chromatography and the relationship between their basicity and RF values. *J. Chromatog.*, **254**, 35-44.

Paalme, L., Uibopuu, H., Rohtla, I., Pahapill, J., Gubergrits, M. & Jacquignon, P.C. (1982) Reactivity of PAH in UV- and γ-radiation initiated oxidation reactions. In: *Polynuclear Hydrocarbons: Formation, Metabolism and Measurement* (Proceedings of the 7th International Symposium, Columbus, Ohio), Columbus, OH, Battelle Press, pp. 999-1008.

Parks, W.C., Schurdak, M.E., Randerath, K., Maher, V.M. & McCormick, J.J. (1986) Human cell-mediated cytotoxicity, mutagenicity and DNA adduct formation of 7*H*-dibenzo(*c,g*)carbazole and its *N*-methyl derivative in diploid human fibroblasts. *Cancer Res.*, **46**, 4706-4711.

Perin, F., Dufour, M., Mispelter, J., Ekert, B., Künneke, C., Oesch, F. & Zajdela, F. (1981) Heterocyclic polycyclic aromatic hydrocarbon carcinogenesis: 7H-dibenzo[*c,g*]carbazole metabolism by microsomal enzymes from mouse and rat liver. *Chem.-Biol. Interactions*, **35**, 267-284.

Podaný, V., Vachálková, A., Miertus, S. & Bahna, L. (1975) Electrochemical properties of polycyclic compounds studied by the polarographic method in anhydrous systems. II. Polarographic study of carcinogenic nitrogen compounds in dimethylformamide and comparison of half-wave potentials with quantum-chemical calculations of molecular orbitals. *Neoplasma*, **22**, 469-482.

Podaný, V., Vachálková, A. & Bahna, L. (1976) Electrochemical properties of polycyclic compounds studied by a polarographic method in anhydrous systems. III. Polarographic reduction potentials of carcinogenic nitrogen compounds in dimethylsulfoxide. *Neoplasma*, **23**, 617-622.

Pouchert, C.J., ed. (1970) *The Aldrich Library of Infrared Spectra*, Milwaukee, WI, Aldrich Chemical Company, p. 1011.

Robinson, D.A. (1973) Benzacridine and condensed acridines. In: Acheson, R.M., ed., *Acridines*, 2nd ed., New York, Interscience, pp. 547-565.

Rostad, C.E. & Pereira, W.E. (1986) Kovats and Lee retention indices determined by gas chromatography/mass spectrometry for organic compounds of environmental interest. *J. High Res. Chromatog. Chromatog. Comm.*, **9**, 328-334.

Royal Society of Chemistry (1983a) *Eight Peak Index of Mass Spectra*, Vol. 1, Part 2, London, p. 752.

Royal Society of Chemistry (1983b) *Eight Peak Index of Mass Spectra*, Vol. 1, Part 2, London, p. 794.

Saito, N., Tanaka, C. & Okubo, M. (1956) Studies on the reaction of formamide. I. Reactions of formamide on the phenolic hydroxyl groups. *J. Pharm. Soc. Jap.*, **76**, 359-361.

Sârbu, C., Horn, M. & Marutoiu, C. (1983) Dünnschichtchromatographische Nachweismethoden für Dicarbonsäuren. *J. Chromatog.*, **281**, 345-347.

Schoen, J. & Bogdanowicz, K. (1960) The condensation of N,N′-di-naphthylthiourea with alicyclic ketones. Synthesis of compounds of the type 9-(β-naphthylamino)-benzo-hydroacridine. *Roczniki Chemii*, **34**, 1339-1346.

Schoen, J. & Laskowska, W. (1965) Condensation of N,N′-diaryl-derivatives of thiourea with β-tetralone. Synthesis of compounds of the type 1,2-benzo- and 1,2:7,8-dibenzo-3,4-dihydroacridine. *Roczniki Chemii, Ann. Soc. Chim. Polonorum*, **39**, 1633-1644.

Schoental, R. & Scott, E.J.Y. (1949) Fluorescence spectra of polycyclic aromatic hydrocarbons in solution. *J. Chem. Soc.*, 1683-1696.

Schronk, L.R., Grisby, R.D. & Hanks, A.R. (1981) Reversed phase HPLC retention behavior of coal related nitrogen heterocyclic compounds. *J. Chromatog. Sci.*, **19**, 490-495.

Senier, A. & Austin, P.C. (1906) Dinaphthacridines. *J. Chem. Soc.*, **89**, 1387-1399.

Senier, A. & Goodwin, W. (1902) The action of methylene diiodide on aryl- and naphthyl-amines: Diarylmethylenediamines, acridines and naphthacridines. *J. Chem. Soc.*, **81**, 280-290.

Shinohara, R., Kido, A., Okamoto, Y. & Takeshita, R. (1983) Determination of azaarenes in water by gas chromatography and gas chromatography-mass spectrometry. *J. Chromatog.*, **256**, 81-91.

Sigvardson, K.W., Kennish, J.M. & Birks, J.W. (1984) Peroxyoxalate chemiluminescence detection of polycyclic aromatic amines in liquid chromatography. *Analyt. Chem.*, **56**, 1096-1102.

Uibopuu, H.M., Vodzinkski, Y.U., Tikhova, N.Y., Kirso, U.E. & Jacquignon, P.C. (1987) Polynuclear heterocyclic hydrocarbons. I. Electrooxidation at graphite electrode. *J. Gen. Chem.* **57**, 1379-1382.

Ullmann, F. & Fetvadjian, A. (1903) Ueber Dinaphtacridine. *Chem. Ber.*, **36**, 1027-1031.

Van Duuren, B.L., Bilbao, J.A. & Joseph, C.A. (1960) The carcinogenic nitrogen heterocyclics in cigarette-smoke condensate. *J. Natl. Cancer Inst.*, **25**, 53-61.

Warshawsky, D. & Myers, B.L. (1981) The metabolism of 7H-dibenzo[c,g]carbazole, an N-heterocyclic aromatic, in the isolated perfused lung. *Cancer Lett.*, **12**, 153-159.

Wilson, B.W., Pelroy, R.A., Mahlum, D.D., Frazier, M.E., Later, D.W. & Wright, C.W. (1984) Comparative chemical composition and biological activity of single- and two-stage coal liquefaction process stream. *Fuel*, **63**, 56-55.

Woo, C.S., D'Silva, A.P. & Fassel, V.A. (1980) Characterization of environmental samples for polynuclear aromatic hydrocarbons by an X-ray excited optical luminescence technique. *Analyt. Chem.*, **52**, 159-164.

Wright, C.W., Later, D.W., Pelroy, R.A., Mahlum, D.D. & Wilson, B.W. (1985) Comparative chemical and biological analysis of coal tar-based therapeutic agents to other coal-derived materials. *J. Appl. Toxicol.*, **5**, 80-88.

PUBLICATIONS OF THE INTERNATIONAL
AGENCY FOR RESEARCH ON CANCER
Scientific Publications Series

(Available from Oxford University Press through local bookshops)

No. 1 Liver Cancer
1971; 176 pages (*out of print*)

No. 2 Oncogenesis and Herpesviruses
Edited by P.M. Biggs, G. de-Thé and L.N. Payne
1972; 515 pages (*out of print*)

No. 3 N-Nitroso Compounds: Analysis and Formation
Edited by P. Bogovski, R. Preussman and E.A. Walker
1972; 140 pages (*out of print*)

No. 4 Transplacental Carcinogenesis
Edited by L. Tomatis and U. Mohr
1973; 181 pages (*out of print*)

No. 5/6 Pathology of Tumours in Laboratory Animals, Volume 1, Tumours of the Rat
Edited by V.S. Turusov
1973/1976; 533 pages; £50.00

No. 7 Host Environment Interactions in the Etiology of Cancer in Man
Edited by R. Doll and I. Vodopija
1973; 464 pages; £32.50

No. 8 Biological Effects of Asbestos
Edited by P. Bogovski, J.C. Gilson, V. Timbrell and J.C. Wagner
1973; 346 pages (*out of print*)

No. 9 N-Nitroso Compounds in the Environment
Edited by P. Bogovski and E.A. Walker
1974; 243 pages; £21.00

No. 10 Chemical Carcinogenesis Essays
Edited by R. Montesano and L. Tomatis
1974; 230 pages (*out of print*)

No. 11 Oncogenesis and Herpesviruses II
Edited by G. de-Thé, M.A. Epstein and H. zur Hausen
1975; Part I: 511 pages
Part II: 403 pages; £65.00

No. 12 Screening Tests in Chemical Carcinogenesis
Edited by R. Montesano, H. Bartsch and L. Tomatis
1976; 666 pages; £45.00

No. 13 Environmental Pollution and Carcinogenic Risks
Edited by C. Rosenfeld and W. Davis
1975; 441 pages (*out of print*)

No. 14 Environmental N-Nitroso Compounds. Analysis and Formation
Edited by E.A. Walker, P. Bogovski and L. Griciute
1976; 512 pages; £37.50

No. 15 Cancer Incidence in Five Continents, Volume III
Edited by J.A.H. Waterhouse, C. Muir, P. Correa and J. Powell
1976; 584 pages; (*out of print*)

No. 16 Air Pollution and Cancer in Man
Edited by U. Mohr, D. Schmähl and L. Tomatis
1977; 328 pages (*out of print*)

No. 17 Directory of On-going Research in Cancer Epidemiology 1977
Edited by C.S. Muir and G. Wagner
1977; 599 pages (*out of print*)

No. 18 Environmental Carcinogens. Selected Methods of Analysis. Volume 1: Analysis of Volatile Nitrosamines in Food
Editor-in-Chief: H. Egan
1978; 212 pages (*out of print*)

No. 19 Environmental Aspects of N-Nitroso Compounds
Edited by E.A. Walker, M. Castegnaro, L. Griciute and R.E. Lyle
1978; 561 pages (*out of print*)

No. 20 Nasopharyngeal Carcinoma: Etiology and Control
Edited by G. de-Thé and Y. Ito
1978; 606 pages (*out of print*)

No. 21 Cancer Registration and its Techniques
Edited by R. MacLennan, C. Muir, R. Steinitz and A. Winkler
1978; 235 pages; £35.00

No. 22 Environmental Carcinogens. Selected Methods of Analysis. Volume 2: Methods for the Measurement of Vinyl Chloride in Poly(vinyl chloride), Air, Water and Foodstuffs
Editor-in-Chief: H. Egan
1978; 142 pages (*out of print*)

No. 23 Pathology of Tumours in Laboratory Animals. Volume II: Tumours of the Mouse
Editor-in-Chief: V.S. Turusov
1979; 669 pages (*out of print*)

No. 24 Oncogenesis and Herpesviruses III
Edited by G. de-Thé, W. Henle and F. Rapp
1978; Part I: 580 pages, Part II: 512 pages (*out of print*)

Prices, valid for September 1991, are subject to change without notice

No. 25 **Carcinogenic Risk. Strategies for Intervention**
Edited by W. Davis and
C. Rosenfeld
1979; 280 pages (*out of print*)

No. 26 **Directory of On-going Research in Cancer Epidemiology 1978**
Edited by C.S. Muir and G. Wagner
1978; 550 pages (*out of print*)

No. 27 **Molecular and Cellular Aspects of Carcinogen Screening Tests**
Edited by R. Montesano,
H. Bartsch and L. Tomatis
1980; 372 pages; £29.00

No. 28 **Directory of On-going Research in Cancer Epidemiology 1979**
Edited by C.S. Muir and G. Wagner
1979; 672 pages (*out of print*)

No. 29 **Environmental Carcinogens. Selected Methods of Analysis. Volume 3: Analysis of Polycyclic Aromatic Hydrocarbons in Environmental Samples**
Editor-in-Chief: H. Egan
1979; 240 pages (*out of print*)

No. 30 **Biological Effects of Mineral Fibres**
Editor-in-Chief: J.C. Wagner
1980; **Volume 1:** 494 pages; **Volume 2:** 513 pages; £65.00

No. 31 *N*-**Nitroso Compounds: Analysis, Formation and Occurrence**
Edited by E.A. Walker, L. Griciute,
M. Castegnaro and M. Börzsönyi
1980; 835 pages (*out of print*)

No. 32 **Statistical Methods in Cancer Research. Volume 1. The Analysis of Case-control Studies**
By N.E. Breslow and N.E. Day
1980; 338 pages; £20.00

No. 33 **Handling Chemical Carcinogens in the Laboratory**
Edited by R. Montesano *et al.*
1979; 32 pages (*out of print*)

No. 34 **Pathology of Tumours in Laboratory Animals. Volume III. Tumours of the Hamster**
Editor-in-Chief: V.S. Turusov
1982; 461 pages; £39.00

No. 35 **Directory of On-going Research in Cancer Epidemiology 1980**
Edited by C.S. Muir and G. Wagner
1980; 660 pages (*out of print*)

No. 36 **Cancer Mortality by Occupation and Social Class 1851-1971**
Edited by W.P.D. Logan
1982; 253 pages; £22.50

No. 37 **Laboratory Decontamination and Destruction of Aflatoxins B$_1$, B$_2$, G$_1$, G$_2$ in Laboratory Wastes**
Edited by M. Castegnaro *et al.*
1980; 56 pages; £6.50

No. 38 **Directory of On-going Research in Cancer Epidemiology 1981**
Edited by C.S. Muir and G. Wagner
1981; 696 pages (*out of print*)

No. 39 **Host Factors in Human Carcinogenesis**
Edited by H. Bartsch and
B. Armstrong
1982; 583 pages; £46.00

No. 40 **Environmental Carcinogens. Selected Methods of Analysis. Volume 4: Some Aromatic Amines and Azo Dyes in the General and Industrial Environment**
Edited by L. Fishbein,
M. Castegnaro, I.K. O'Neill and
H. Bartsch
1981; 347 pages; £29.00

No. 41 *N*-**Nitroso Compounds: Occurrence and Biological Effects**
Edited by H. Bartsch, I.K. O'Neill,
M. Castegnaro and M. Okada
1982; 755 pages; £48.00

No. 42 **Cancer Incidence in Five Continents, Volume IV**
Edited by J. Waterhouse, C. Muir,
K. Shanmugaratnam and J. Powell
1982; 811 pages (*out of print*)

No. 43 **Laboratory Decontamination and Destruction of Carcinogens in Laboratory Wastes: Some *N*-Nitrosamines**
Edited by M. Castegnaro *et al.*
1982; 73 pages; £7.50

No. 44 **Environmental Carcinogens. Selected Methods of Analysis. Volume 5: Some Mycotoxins**
Edited by L. Stoloff, M. Castegnaro,
P. Scott, I.K. O'Neill and H. Bartsch
1983; 455 pages; £29.00

No. 45 **Environmental Carcinogens. Selected Methods of Analysis. Volume 6: *N*-Nitroso Compounds**
Edited by R. Preussmann, I.K.
O'Neill, G. Eisenbrand, B.
Spiegelhalder and H. Bartsch
1983; 508 pages; £29.00

No. 46 **Directory of On-going Research in Cancer Epidemiology 1982**
Edited by C.S. Muir and G. Wagner
1982; 722 pages (*out of print*)

No. 47 **Cancer Incidence in Singapore 1968–1977**
Edited by K. Shanmugaratnam,
H.P. Lee and N.E. Day
1983; 171 pages (*out of print*)

No. 48 **Cancer Incidence in the USSR (2nd Revised Edition)**
Edited by N.P. Napalkov,
G.F. Tserkovny, V.M. Merabishvili,
D.M. Parkin, M. Smans and
C.S. Muir
1983; 75 pages; £12.00

No. 49 **Laboratory Decontamination and Destruction of Carcinogens in Laboratory Wastes: Some Polycyclic Aromatic Hydrocarbons**
Edited by M. Castegnaro *et al.*
1983; 87 pages; £9.00

No. 50 **Directory of On-going Research in Cancer Epidemiology 1983**
Edited by C.S. Muir and G. Wagner
1983; 731 pages (*out of print*)

No. 51 **Modulators of Experimental Carcinogenesis**
Edited by V. Turusov and R.
Montesano
1983; 307 pages; £22.50

No. 52 **Second Cancers in Relation to Radiation Treatment for Cervical Cancer: Results of a Cancer Registry Collaboration**
Edited by N.E. Day and J.C. Boice, Jr
1984; 207 pages; £20.00

No. 53 **Nickel in the Human Environment**
Editor-in-Chief: F.W. Sunderman, Jr
1984; 529 pages; £41.00

No. 54 **Laboratory Decontamination and Destruction of Carcinogens in Laboratory Wastes: Some Hydrazines**
Edited by M. Castegnaro et al.
1983; 87 pages; £9.00

No. 55 **Laboratory Decontamination and Destruction of Carcinogens in Laboratory Wastes: Some N-Nitrosamides**
Edited by M. Castegnaro et al.
1984; 66 pages; £7.50

No. 56 **Models, Mechanisms and Etiology of Tumour Promotion**
Edited by M. Börzsönyi, N.E. Day, K. Lapis and H. Yamasaki
1984; 532 pages; £42.00

No. 57 *N-Nitroso Compounds:* **Occurrence, Biological Effects and Relevance to Human Cancer**
Edited by I.K. O'Neill, R.C. von Borstel, C.T. Miller, J. Long and H. Bartsch
1984; 1013 pages; £80.00

No. 58 **Age-related Factors in Carcinogenesis**
Edited by A. Likhachev, V. Anisimov and R. Montesano
1985; 288 pages; £20.00

No. 59 **Monitoring Human Exposure to Carcinogenic and Mutagenic Agents**
Edited by A. Berlin, M. Draper, K. Hemminki and H. Vainio
1984; 457 pages; £27.50

No. 60 **Burkitt's Lymphoma: A Human Cancer Model**
Edited by G. Lenoir, G. O'Conor and C.L.M. Olweny
1985; 484 pages; £29.00

No. 61 **Laboratory Decontamination and Destruction of Carcinogens in Laboratory Wastes: Some Haloethers**
Edited by M. Castegnaro et al.
1985; 55 pages; £7.50

No. 62 **Directory of On-going Research in Cancer Epidemiology 1984**
Edited by C.S. Muir and G. Wagner
1984; 717 pages (*out of print*)

No. 63 **Virus-associated Cancers in Africa**
Edited by A.O. Williams, G.T. O'Conor, G.B. de-Thé and C.A. Johnson
1984; 773 pages; £22.00

No. 64 **Laboratory Decontamination and Destruction of Carcinogens in Laboratory Wastes: Some Aromatic Amines and 4-Nitrobiphenyl**
Edited by M. Castegnaro et al.
1985; 84 pages; £6.95

No. 65 **Interpretation of Negative Epidemiological Evidence for Carcinogenicity**
Edited by N.J. Wald and R. Doll
1985; 232 pages; £20.00

No. 66 **The Role of the Registry in Cancer Control**
Edited by D.M. Parkin, G. Wagner and C.S. Muir
1985; 152 pages; £10.00

No. 67 **Transformation Assay of Established Cell Lines: Mechanisms and Application**
Edited by T. Kakunaga and H. Yamasaki
1985; 225 pages; £20.00

No. 68 **Environmental Carcinogens. Selected Methods of Analysis. Volume 7. Some Volatile Halogenated Hydrocarbons**
Edited by L. Fishbein and I.K. O'Neill
1985; 479 pages; £42.00

No. 69 **Directory of On-going Research in Cancer Epidemiology 1985**
Edited by C.S. Muir and G. Wagner
1985; 745 pages; £22.00

No. 70 **The Role of Cyclic Nucleic Acid Adducts in Carcinogenesis and Mutagenesis**
Edited by B. Singer and H. Bartsch
1986; 467 pages; £40.00

No. 71 **Environmental Carcinogens. Selected Methods of Analysis. Volume 8: Some Metals: As, Be, Cd, Cr, Ni, Pb, Se Zn**
Edited by I.K. O'Neill, P. Schuller and L. Fishbein
1986; 485 pages; £42.00

No. 72 **Atlas of Cancer in Scotland, 1975–1980. Incidence and Epidemiological Perspective**
Edited by I. Kemp, P. Boyle, M. Smans and C.S. Muir
1985; 285 pages; £35.00

No. 73 **Laboratory Decontamination and Destruction of Carcinogens in Laboratory Wastes: Some Antineoplastic Agents**
Edited by M. Castegnaro et al.
1985; 163 pages; £10.00

No. 74 **Tobacco: A Major International Health Hazard**
Edited by D. Zaridze and R. Peto
1986; 324 pages; £20.00

No. 75 **Cancer Occurrence in Developing Countries**
Edited by D.M. Parkin
1986; 339 pages; £20.00

No. 76 **Screening for Cancer of the Uterine Cervix**
Edited by M. Hakama, A.B. Miller and N.E. Day
1986; 315 pages; £25.00

No. 77 Hexachlorobenzene: Proceedings of an International Symposium
Edited by C.R. Morris and J.R.P. Cabral
1986; 668 pages; £50.00

No. 78 Carcinogenicity of Alkylating Cytostatic Drugs
Edited by D. Schmähl and J.M. Kaldor
1986; 337 pages; £25.00

No. 79 Statistical Methods in Cancer Research. Volume III: The Design and Analysis of Long-term Animal Experiments
By J.J. Gart, D. Krewski, P.N. Lee, R.E. Tarone and J. Wahrendorf
1986; 213 pages; £20.00

No. 80 Directory of On-going Research in Cancer Epidemiology 1986
Edited by C.S. Muir and G. Wagner
1986; 805 pages; £22.00

No. 81 Environmental Carcinogens: Methods of Analysis and Exposure Measurement. Volume 9: Passive Smoking
Edited by I.K. O'Neill, K.D. Brunnemann, B. Dodet and D. Hoffmann
1987; 383 pages; £35.00

No. 82 Statistical Methods in Cancer Research. Volume II: The Design and Analysis of Cohort Studies
By N.E. Breslow and N.E. Day
1987; 404 pages; £30.00

No. 83 Long-term and Short-term Assays for Carcinogens: A Critical Appraisal
Edited by R. Montesano, H. Bartsch, H. Vainio, J. Wilbourn and H. Yamasaki
1986; 575 pages; £48.00

No. 84 The Relevance of *N*-Nitroso Compounds to Human Cancer: Exposure and Mechanisms
Edited by H. Bartsch, I.K. O'Neill and R. Schulte-Hermann
1987; 671 pages; £50.00

No. 85 Environmental Carcinogens: Methods of Analysis and Exposure Measurement. Volume 10: Benzene and Alkylated Benzenes
Edited by L. Fishbein and I.K. O'Neill
1988; 327 pages; £35.00

No. 86 Directory of On-going Research in Cancer Epidemiology 1987
Edited by D.M. Parkin and J. Wahrendorf
1987; 676 pages; £22.00

No. 87 International Incidence of Childhood Cancer
Edited by D.M. Parkin, C.A. Stiller, C.A. Bieber, G.J. Draper, B. Terracini and J.L. Young
1988; 401 pages; £35.00

No. 88 Cancer Incidence in Five Continents Volume V
Edited by C. Muir, J. Waterhouse, T. Mack, J. Powell and S. Whelan
1987; 1004 pages; £50.00

No. 89 Method for Detecting DNA Damaging Agents in Humans: Applications in Cancer Epidemiology and Prevention
Edited by H. Bartsch, K. Hemminki and I.K. O'Neill
1988; 518 pages; £45.00

No. 90 Non-occupational Exposure to Mineral Fibres
Edited by J. Bignon, J. Peto and R. Saracci
1989; 500 pages; £45.00

No. 91 Trends in Cancer Incidence in Singapore 1968–1982
Edited by H.P. Lee , N.E. Day and K. Shanmugaratnam
1988; 160 pages; £25.00

No. 92 Cell Differentiation, Genes and Cancer
Edited by T. Kakunaga, T. Sugimura, L. Tomatis and H. Yamasaki
1988; 204 pages; £25.00

No. 93 Directory of On-going Research in Cancer Epidemiology 1988
Edited by M. Coleman and J. Wahrendorf
1988; 662 pages (*out of print*)

No. 94 Human Papillomavirus and Cervical Cancer
Edited by N. Muñoz, F.X. Bosch and O.M. Jensen
1989; 154 pages; £19.00

No. 95 Cancer Registration: Principles and Methods
Edited by O.M. Jensen, D.M. Parkin, R. MacLennan, C.S. Muir and R. Skeet
1991; 288 pages; £28.00

No. 96 Perinatal and Multigeneration Carcinogenesis
Edited by N.P. Napalkov, J.M. Rice, L. Tomatis and H. Yamasaki
1989; 436 pages; £48.00

No. 97 Occupational Exposure to Silica and Cancer Risk
Edited by L. Simonato, A.C. Fletcher, R. Saracci and T. Thomas
1990; 124 pages; £19.00

No. 98 Cancer Incidence in Jewish Migrants to Israel, 1961–1981
Edited by R. Steinitz, D.M. Parkin, J.L. Young, C.A. Bieber and L. Katz
1989; 320 pages; £30.00

No. 99 Pathology of Tumours in Laboratory Animals, Second Edition, Volume 1, Tumours of the Rat
Edited by V.S. Turusov and U. Mohr
740 pages; £85.00

No. 100 Cancer: Causes, Occurrence and Control
Editor-in-Chief L. Tomatis
1990; 352 pages; £24.00

No. 101 **Directory of On-going Research in Cancer Epidemiology 1989/90**
Edited by M. Coleman and
J. Wahrendorf
1989; 818 pages; £36.00

No. 102 **Patterns of Cancer in Five Continents**
Edited by S.L. Whelan and
D.M. Parkin
1990; 162 pages; £25.00

No. 103 **Evaluating Effectiveness of Primary Prevention of Cancer**
Edited by M. Hakama, V. Beral, J.W. Cullen and D.M. Parkin
1990; 250 pages; £32.00

No. 104 **Complex Mixtures and Cancer Risk**
Edited by H. Vainio, M. Sorsa and
A.J. McMichael
1990; 442 pages; £38.00

No. 105 **Relevance to Human Cancer of *N*-Nitroso Compounds, Tobacco Smoke and Mycotoxins**
Edited by I.K. O'Neill, J. Chen and
H. Bartsch
1991; 614 pages; £70.00

No. 106 **Atlas of Cancer Incidence in the German Democratic Republic**
Edited by W.H. Mehnert, M. Smans and C.S. Muir
Publ. due 1992; c.328 pages; £42.00

No. 107 **Atlas of Cancer Mortality in the European Economic Community**
Edited by M. Smans, C.S. Muir and
P. Boyle
Publ. due 1991; approx. 230 pages;
£35.00

No. 108 **Environmental Carcinogens: Methods of Analysis and Exposure Measurement. Volume 11: Polychlorinated Dioxins and Dibenzofurans**
Edited by C. Rappe, H.R. Buser,
B. Dodet and I.K. O'Neill
1991; 426 pages; £45.00

No. 109 **Environmental Carcinogens: Methods of Analysis and Exposure Measurement. Volume 12: Indoor Air Contaminants**
Edited by B. Seifert, B. Dodet and
I.K. O'Neill
Publ. due 1992; approx. 400 pages

No. 110 **Directory of On-going Research in Cancer Epidemiology 1991**
Edited by M. Coleman and
J. Wahrendorf
1991; 753 pages; £38.00

No. 111 **Pathology of Tumours in Laboratory Animals, Second Edition, Volume 2, Tumours of the Mouse**
Edited by V.S. Turusov and
U. Mohr
Publ. due 1992; approx. 500 pages

No. 112 **Autopsy in Epidemiology and Medical Research**
Edited by E. Riboli and M. Delendi
1991; 288 pages; £25.00

No. 113 **Laboratory Decontamination and Destruction of Carcinogens in Laboratory Wastes: Some Mycotoxins**
Edited by M. Castegnaro, J. Barek,
J.–M. Frémy, M. Lafontaine,
M. Miraglia, E.B. Sansone and
G.M. Telling
1991; approx. 60 pages; £11.00

No. 114 **Laboratory Decontamination and Destruction of Carcinogens in Laboratory Wastes: Some Polycyclic Heterocyclic Hydrocarbons**
Edited by M. Castegnaro, J. Barek,
J. Jacob, U. Kirso, M. Lafontaine,
E.B. Sansone, G.M. Telling and
T. Vu Duc
1991; approx. 40 pages; £8.00

IARC MONOGRAPHS ON THE EVALUATION OF CARCINOGENIC RISKS TO HUMANS

(Available from booksellers through the network of WHO Sales Agents)

Volume 1 **Some Inorganic Substances, Chlorinated Hydrocarbons, Aromatic Amines, N-Nitroso Compounds, and Natural Products**
1972; 184 pages (*out of print*)

Volume 2 **Some Inorganic and Organometallic Compounds**
1973; 181 pages (out of print)

Volume 3 **Certain Polycyclic Aromatic Hydrocarbons and Heterocyclic Compounds**
1973; 271 pages (*out of print*)

Volume 4 **Some Aromatic Amines, Hydrazine and Related Substances, N-Nitroso Compounds and Miscellaneous Alkylating Agents**
1974; 286 pages;
Sw. fr. 18.-/US $14.40

Volume 5 **Some Organochlorine Pesticides**
1974; 241 pages (*out of print*)

Volume 6 **Sex Hormones**
1974; 243 pages (*out of print*)

Volume 7 **Some Anti-Thyroid and Related Substances, Nitrofurans and Industrial Chemicals**
1974; 326 pages (*out of print*)

Volume 8 **Some Aromatic Azo Compounds**
1975; 375 pages;
Sw. fr. 36.-/US $28.80

Volume 9 **Some Aziridines, N-, S- and O-Mustards and Selenium**
1975; 268 pages;
Sw.fr. 27.-/US $21.60

Volume 10 **Some Naturally Occurring Substances**
1976; 353 pages (*out of print*)

Volume 11 **Cadmium, Nickel, Some Epoxides, Miscellaneous Industrial Chemicals and General Considerations on Volatile Anaesthetics**
1976; 306 pages (*out of print*)

Volume 12 **Some Carbamates, Thiocarbamates and Carbazides**
1976; 282 pages;
Sw. fr. 34.-/US $27.20

Volume 13 **Some Miscellaneous Pharmaceutical Substances**
1977; 255 pages;
Sw. fr. 30.-/US$ 24.00

Volume 14 **Asbestos**
1977; 106 pages (*out of print*)

Volume 15 **Some Fumigants, The Herbicides 2,4-D and 2,4,5-T, Chlorinated Dibenzodioxins and Miscellaneous Industrial Chemicals**
1977; 354 pages;
Sw. fr. 50.-/US $40.00

Volume 16 **Some Aromatic Amines and Related Nitro Compounds - Hair Dyes, Colouring Agents and Miscellaneous Industrial Chemicals**
1978; 400 pages;
Sw. fr. 50.-/US $40.00

Volume 17 **Some N-Nitroso Compounds**
1987; 365 pages;
Sw. fr. 50.-/US $40.00

Volume 18 **Polychlorinated Biphenyls and Polybrominated Biphenyls**
1978; 140 pages;
Sw. fr. 20.-/US $16.00

Volume 19 **Some Monomers, Plastics and Synthetic Elastomers, and Acrolein**
1979; 513 pages;
Sw. fr. 60.-/US $48.00

Volume 20 **Some Halogenated Hydrocarbons**
1979; 609 pages (*out of print*)

Volume 21 **Sex Hormones (II)**
1979; 583 pages;
Sw. fr. 60.-/US $48.00

Volume 22 **Some Non-Nutritive Sweetening Agents**
1980; 208 pages;
Sw. fr. 25.-/US $20.00

Volume 23 **Some Metals and Metallic Compounds**
1980; 438 pages (*out of print*)

Volume 24 **Some Pharmaceutical Drugs**
1980; 337 pages;
Sw. fr. 40.-/US $32.00

Volume 25 **Wood, Leather and Some Associated Industries**
1981; 412 pages;
Sw. fr. 60.-/US $48.00

Volume 26 **Some Antineoplastic and Immunosuppressive Agents**
1981; 411 pages;
Sw. fr. 62.-/US $49.60

Volume 27 **Some Aromatic Amines, Anthraquinones and Nitroso Compounds, and Inorganic Fluorides Used in Drinking Water and Dental Preparations**
1982; 341 pages;
Sw. fr. 40.-/US $32.00

Volume 28 **The Rubber Industry**
1982; 486 pages;
Sw. fr. 70.-/US $56.00

Volume 29 **Some Industrial Chemicals and Dyestuffs**
1982; 416 pages;
Sw. fr. 60.-/US $48.00

Volume 30 **Miscellaneous Pesticides**
1983; 424 pages;
Sw. fr. 60.-/US $48.00

Volume 31 **Some Food Additives, Feed Additives and Naturally Occurring Substances**
1983; 314 pages;
Sw. fr. 60-/US $48.00

Volume 32 Polynuclear Aromatic
Compounds, Part 1: Chemical,
Environmental and Experimental
Data
1984; 477 pages;
Sw. fr. 60.-/US $48.00

Volume 33 Polynuclear Aromatic
Compounds, Part 2: Carbon Blacks,
Mineral Oils and Some Nitroarenes
1984; 245 pages;
Sw. fr. 50.-/US $40.00

Volume 34 Polynuclear Aromatic
Compounds, Part 3: Industrial
Exposures in Aluminium
Production, Coal Gasification, Coke
Production, and Iron and Steel
Founding
1984; 219 pages;
Sw. fr. 48.-/US $38.40

Volume 35 Polynuclear Aromatic
Compounds, Part 4: Bitumens,
Coal-tars and Derived Products,
Shale-oils and Soots
1985; 271 pages;
Sw. fr. 70.-/US $56.00

Volume 36 Allyl Compounds,
Aldehydes, Epoxides and Peroxides
1985; 369 pages;
Sw. fr. 70.-/US $70.00

Volume 37 Tobacco Habits Other
than Smoking: Betel-quid and
Areca-nut Chewing; and some
Related Nitrosamines
1985; 291 pages;
Sw. fr. 70.-/US $56.00

Volume 38 Tobacco Smoking
1986; 421 pages;
Sw. fr. 75.-/US $60.00

Volume 39 Some Chemicals Used in
Plastics and Elastomers
1986; 403 pages;
Sw. fr. 60.-/US $48.00

Volume 40 Some Naturally
Occurring and Synthetic Food
Components, Furocoumarins and
Ultraviolet Radiation
1986; 444 pages;
Sw. fr. 65.-/US $52.00

Volume 41 Some Halogenated
Hydrocarbons and Pesticide
Exposures
1986; 434 pages;
Sw. fr. 65.-/US $52.00

Volume 42 Silica and Some Silicates
1987; 289 pages;
Sw. fr. 65.-/US $52.00

Volume 43 Man-Made Mineral
Fibres and Radon
1988; 300 pages;
Sw. fr. 65.-/US $52.00

Volume 44 Alcohol Drinking
1988; 416 pages;
Sw. fr. 65.-/US $52.00

Volume 45 Occupational Exposures
in Petroleum Refining; Crude Oil
and Major Petroleum Fuels
1989; 322 pages;
Sw. fr. 65.-/US $52.00

Volume 46 Diesel and Gasoline
Engine Exhausts and Some
Nitroarenes
1989; 458 pages;
Sw. fr. 65.-/US $52.00

Volume 47 Some Organic Solvents,
Resin Monomers and Related
Compounds, Pigments and
Occupational Exposures in Paint
Manufacture and Painting
1990; 536 pages;
Sw. fr. 85.-/US $68.00

Volume 48 Some Flame Retardants
and Textile Chemicals, and
Exposures in the Textile
Manufacturing Industry
1990; 345 pages;
Sw. fr. 65.-/US $52.00

Volume 49 Chromium, Nickel and
Welding
1990; 677 pages;
Sw. fr. 95.-/US$76.00

Volume 50 Pharmaceutical Drugs
1990; 415 pages;
Sw. fr. 65.-/US$52.00

Volume 51 Coffee, Tea, Mate,
Methylxanthines and Methylglyoxal
1991; 513 pages;
Sw. fr. 80.-/US$64.00

Volume 52 Chlorinated
Drinking-water; Chlorination
By-products; Some Other
Halogenated Compounds; Cobalt
and Cobalt Compounds
1991; 544 pages;
Sw. fr. 80.-/US$64.00

Supplement No. 1
Chemicals and Industrial Processes
Associated with Cancer in Humans
(IARC Monographs, Volumes 1 to
20)
1979; 71 pages; (*out of print*)

Supplement No. 2
Long-term and Short-term Screening
Assays for Carcinogens: A Critical
Appraisal
1980; 426 pages;
Sw. fr. 40.-/US $32.00

Supplement No. 3
Cross Index of Synonyms and Trade
Names in Volumes 1 to 26
1982; 199 pages (*out of print*)

Supplement No. 4
Chemicals, Industrial Processes and
Industries Associated with Cancer in
Humans (IARC Monographs,
Volumes 1 to 29)
1982; 292 pages (*out of print*)

Supplement No. 5
Cross Index of Synonyms and Trade
Names in Volumes 1 to 36
1985; 259 pages;
Sw. fr. 46.-/US $36.80

Supplement No. 6
Genetic and Related Effects: An
Updating of Selected IARC
Monographs from Volumes 1 to 42
1987; 729 pages;
Sw. fr. 80.-/US $64.00

Supplement No. 7
Overall Evaluations of
Carcinogenicity: An Updating of
IARC Monographs Volumes 1-42
1987; 434 pages;
Sw. fr. 65.-/US $52.00

Supplement No. 8
Cross Index of Synonyms and Trade
Names in Volumes 1 to 46 of the
IARC Monographs
1990; 260 pages;
Sw. fr. 60.-/US $48.00

IARC TECHNICAL REPORTS*

No. 1 **Cancer in Costa Rica**
Edited by R. Sierra,
R. Barrantes, G. Muñoz Leiva, D.M.
Parkin, C.A. Bieber and
N. Muñoz Calero
1988; 124 pages;
Sw. fr. 30.-/US $24.00

No. 2 **SEARCH: A Computer Package to Assist the Statistical Analysis of Case-control Studies**
Edited by G.J. Macfarlane,
P. Boyle and P. Maisonneuve (in press)

No. 3 **Cancer Registration in the European Economic Community**
Edited by M.P. Coleman and
E. Démaret
1988; 188 pages;
Sw. fr. 30.-/US $24.00

No. 4 **Diet, Hormones and Cancer: Methodological Issues for Prospective Studies**
Edited by E. Riboli and
R. Saracci
1988; 156 pages;
Sw. fr. 30.-/US $24.00

No. 5 **Cancer in the Philippines**
Edited by A.V. Laudico,
D. Esteban and D.M. Parkin
1989; 186 pages;
Sw. fr. 30.-/US $24.00

No. 6 **La genèse du Centre International de Recherche sur le Cancer**
Par R. Sohier et A.G.B. Sutherland
1990; 104 pages
Sw. fr. 30.-/US $24.00

No. 7 **Epidémiologie du cancer dans les pays de langue latine**
1990; 310 pages
Sw. fr. 30.-/US $24.00

No. 8 **Comparative Study of Anti-smoking Legislation in Countries of the European Economic Community**
Edited by A. Sasco
1990; c. 80 pages
Sw. fr. 30.-/US $24.00
(English and French editions available) (in press)

DIRECTORY OF AGENTS BEING TESTED FOR CARCINOGENICITY (Until Vol. 13 Information Bulletin on the Survey of Chemicals Being Tested for Carcinogenicity)*

No. 8 Edited by M.-J. Ghess,
H. Bartsch and L. Tomatis
1979; 604 pages; Sw. fr. 40.-

No. 9 Edited by M.-J. Ghess,
J.D. Wilbourn, H. Bartsch and
L. Tomatis
1981; 294 pages; Sw. fr. 41.-

No. 10 Edited by M.-J. Ghess,
J.D. Wilbourn and H. Bartsch
1982; 362 pages; Sw. fr. 42.-

No. 11 Edited by M.-J. Ghess,
J.D. Wilbourn, H. Vainio and
H. Bartsch
1984; 362 pages; Sw. fr. 50.-

No. 12 Edited by M.-J. Ghess,
J.D. Wilbourn, A. Tossavainen and
H. Vainio
1986; 385 pages; Sw. fr. 50.-

No. 13 Edited by M.-J. Ghess,
J.D. Wilbourn and A. Aitio 1988;
404 pages; Sw. fr. 43.-

No. 14 Edited by M.-J. Ghess,
J.D. Wilbourn and H. Vainio
1990; 370 pages; Sw. fr. 45.-

NON-SERIAL PUBLICATIONS †

Alcool et Cancer
By A. Tuyns (in French only)
1978; 42 pages; Fr. fr. 35.-

Cancer Morbidity and Causes of Death Among Danish Brewery Workers
By O.M. Jensen
1980; 143 pages; Fr. fr. 75.-

Directory of Computer Systems Used in Cancer Registries
By H.R. Menck and D.M. Parkin
1986; 236 pages; Fr. fr. 50.-

* Available from booksellers through the network of WHO sales agents.

† Available directly from IARC

IMPRIMERIE DARANTIERE DIJON-QUETIGNY